BEYOND THE
MEDITERRANEAN DIET

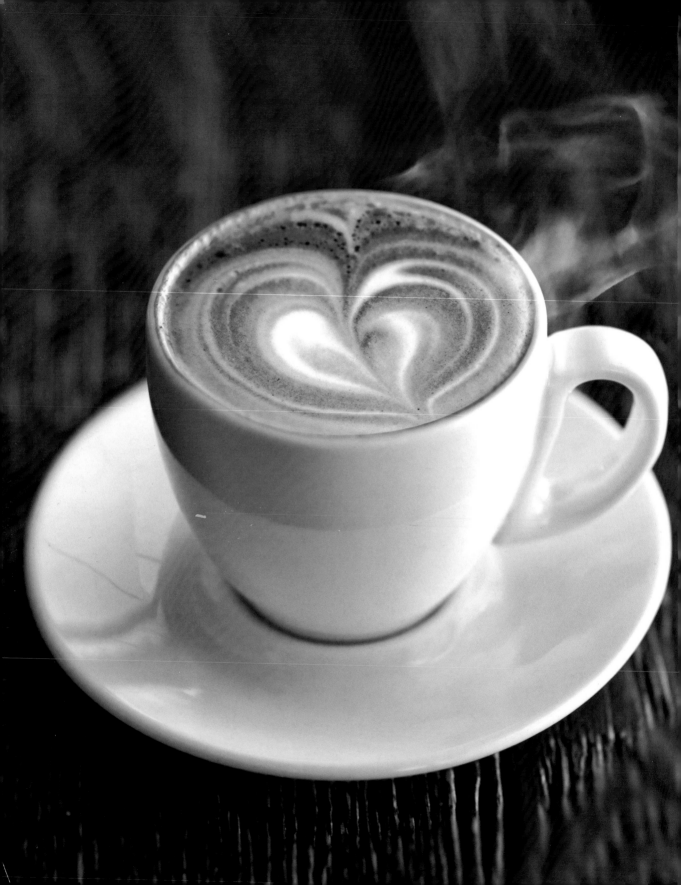

BEYOND THE MEDITERRANEAN DIET

EUROPEAN SECRETS OF THE SUPER-HEALTHY

LAYNE LIEBERMAN, MS, RD, CDN

Internationally Recognized Nutrition Expert

Featuring 50 Mouthwatering and Nutritious Recipes

Foreword by Judith A. Gilbride, PhD, RD, FADA, Professor of Nutrition,
New York University, Past President of the Academy of Nutrition and Dietetics

WorldRD LLC

COLORADO

For information about this title or to order other books and/or electronic media, contact the publisher:

WorldRD LLC

www.WorldRD.com

Layne@WorldRD.com

Library of Congress Control Number: 2013946453

ISBN: 978-0-9891812-1-1

Printed in Canada

Editor: Claire Gerus
Cover and interior design: Bill Greaves
Typesetter: 1106 Design
Indexer: Dan Connolly
Majority of photography: Layne Lieberman

DISCLAIMER

This book and any associated website references are intended to provide general information regarding the subject matter covered. It is not meant to provide any medical opinion, healthcare advice, or to serve as a substitute for the advice of licensed medical professionals. Rather, this information is provided as a resource only and is not to be used or relied on for any diagnostic or treatment purposes. This information does not create any confidential or patient-healthcare professional relationship.

Health, diet and lifestyle have medical consequences and vary from one individual to the next. It is therefore the responsibility of the reader to know whether, and to what extent, this information should be applied in his or her life. Please consult your healthcare provider before making any healthcare decisions or for guidance about a specific medical condition. Layne Lieberman and WorldRD LLC and their respective affiliates expressly disclaim responsibility, and shall have no liability whatsoever, for any direct or indirect damage, loss or injury suffered as a result of your use and/or reliance on the information contained in this publication or affiliated websites or due to any error, inaccuracy or omission.

Layne Lieberman and WorldRD LLC does not endorse any material or organization referenced in the book or on any affiliated websites or otherwise warrant that any information mentioned in the book or on affiliated websites is complete or accurate.

By reading this book or visiting affiliated websites, you understand and agree to the foregoing disclaimer, which may, from time to time, be changed or supplemented by WorldRD LLC.

CREDITS

Any omissions for copyright or credit are unintentional, and appropriate credit will be given in future editions if such copyright holders contact the publisher.

THIS BOOK IS DEDICATED TO:

Michael Liebelson for being my love, rock, soul mate, super-taster,
keen critic and the greatest husband in the world!

Benjamin Anapol and Alexander Anapol for being my ingredient-shoppers,
taste-testers, recipe-testers, photographers and the most awesome sons!

Loretta and David "Fuzzy" Lieberman from Boca Raton, Florida, for being
supportive, caring, loving and outstanding parents throughout my life!

In memory of Dora and Benny Margolies, my European grandparents, for
bringing our family, every Sunday, the freshest fruits and vegetables.
My grandfather owned a produce market in the Bronx, and I will never forget
his big smile as he handed me the juiciest piece of fruit and laughed delightedly
when the juice ran down my face.

I love you all forever!

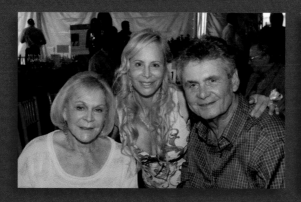 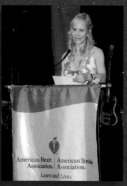

LAYNE'S PARENTS, LORETTA AND DAVID LIEBERMAN, WITH LAYNE AT THE HAMPTONS HEART BALL, JUNE, 2012

LAYNE AT THE PODIUM, AFTER BEING AWARDED THE DISTINGUISHED HEART HEALTH ACHIEVEMENT AWARD,
PRESENTED BY THE AMERICAN HEART ASSOCIATION IN BRIDGEHAMPTON, NY, JUNE 2012.

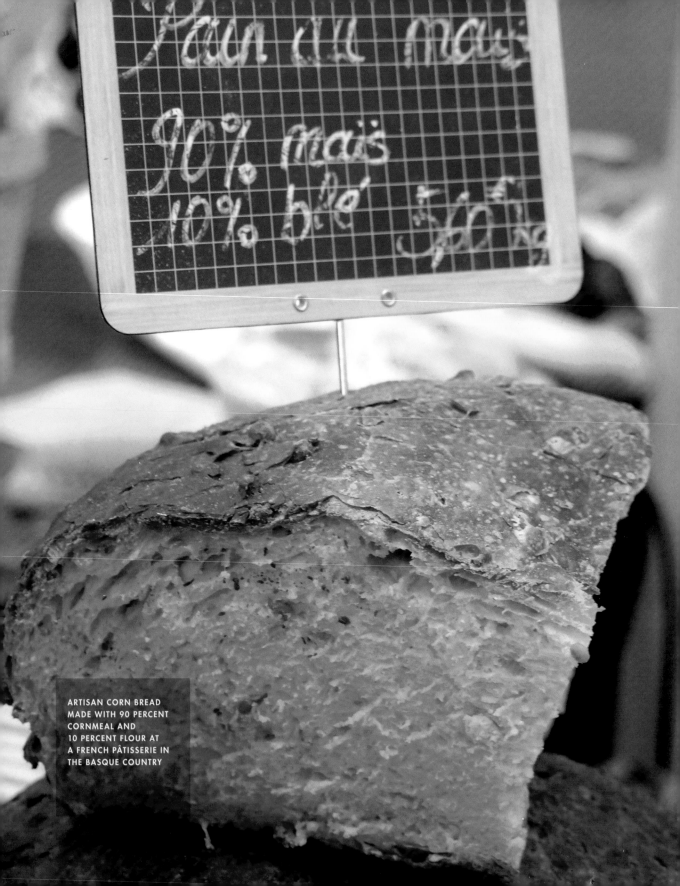

ARTISAN CORN BREAD
MADE WITH 90 PERCENT
CORNMEAL AND
10 PERCENT FLOUR AT
A FRENCH PÂTISSERIE IN
THE BASQUE COUNTRY

TABLE OF CONTENTS

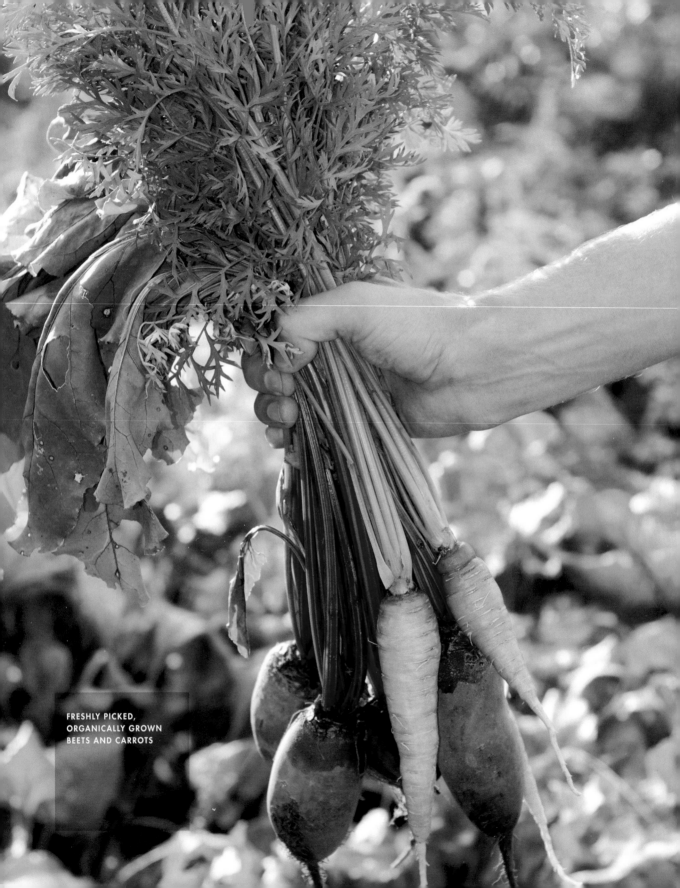

FRESHLY PICKED,
ORGANICALLY GROWN
BEETS AND CARROTS

Welcome to a new culinary worldview, introduced by my dedicated colleague, Layne Lieberman, who made good on her vow to discover why we Americans are facing so many dietary challenges in modern times. Now, in *Beyond the Mediterranean Diet: European Secrets of the Super-Healthy,* Layne reveals the benefits of going beyond the famed "Mediterranean diet" to reach new levels of health, stay slim and enjoy fine food.

For over 20 years, Layne, a former student of mine, has helped her clients choose "healthy" over "convenient" when it comes to making food choices. But as the world became more accustomed to larger portions and the allure of convenience foods, she watched with growing alarm as Americans grew increasingly overweight, and then obese. Today, we are in the midst of an alarming epidemic of heart disease, obesity, diabetes and cancer. Many of these illnesses are linked to today's dietary choices, especially those featuring excessive amounts of sugar, fat, additives and calories.

When Layne discovered that three European countries had a stellar record for longevity, physical well-being, and slim, healthy bodies, she spent two years uncovering their health secrets.

We've all heard of the famous Mediterranean diet. Back in the 1980s, it was a positive introduction to that area's fresh, natural foods. However, it is no longer in keeping with today's fast-moving, "grab, gobble and gulp" lifestyle. Today, the fittest Europeans are choosing sustainable local products and avoiding the temptations of processed and altered food products.

And it couldn't be easier—wherever you live—to follow their example. This book introduces you to the simple steps Europeans follow, such as eating more slowly, choosing smaller portions, and knowing how to shop in both small and large marketplaces. You will discover how to cut down on fat, sugar and sodium, and best of all, you can try Layne's delicious, European-inspired recipes (complete with nutritional analyses), and a variety of low-fat, gluten-free and vegetarian options as well.

Here is a treasure trove of health information, nutritious recipes and a new culinary lifestyle that will bring you the same life-changing results enjoyed by those fortunate enough to live in these top three super-healthy countries!

Enjoy!

Judith A. Gilbride, PhD, RD, FADA

Professor of Nutrition and Dietetics, New York University
Past President, The American Dietetic Association (now the Academy of Nutrition and Dietetics), 2006–2007

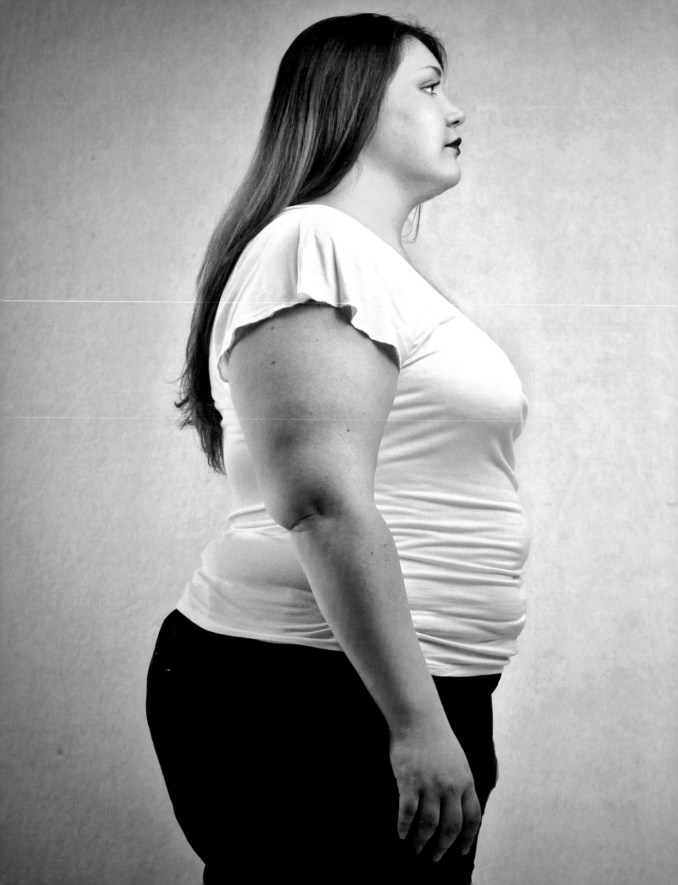

Introduction

WHY WE'RE LOSING THE FIGHT WITH FAT

BEFORE-AND-AFTER
WEIGHT-LOSS PHOTOS
OF A YOUNG WOMAN

L et's not sugarcoat the facts—we're in the midst of an obesity and chronic disease epidemic that's taking a huge toll on world health. Just looking at our own country, a staggering one-third of American adults are obese, while another third are overweight. In fact, it's predicted that the obesity rate in the U.S. could reach 42 percent by 2030!

Even more worrisome is the fact that obesity in American children has jumped from four percent in the early 1980s to nearly 20 percent today! Their life spans are now projected to be shorter than ours will be, along with a higher rate of illness. While hard to imagine that this can happen in our progressive, modern society, numbers don't lie. Even worse, the increasing numbers of obese Americans will lead to more cases of diabetes, hypertension, heart disease and other chronic illnesses.

According to the World Health Organization, America ranks lowest for longevity out of the world's 17 most affluent nations. We also have some of the highest rates of heart disease, obesity and diabetes.

And by the way, we are not talking about just the underserved or economically challenged. Prosperous white Americans die earlier than their international cousins, and even fit, nonsmoking Americans have higher disease rates than do our contemporaries in other affluent countries. This doesn't make sense considering that we spend more on health care per capita than any other nation.

Admittedly, we're increasingly reliant on cars and get less exercise, but that's not our only problem. We also gulp down more calories per person than citizens of other countries. It's significant that America's growing population of immigrants is generally in better health when they arrive here than their native-born American neighbors. But the health of the sons and daughters of these immigrants soon declines to that of other Americans. It's clear that our lifestyle, from how much we eat to how little we exercise, is reducing out longevity relative to other affluent countries.

Why is America losing the obesity battle? For years, we've had several hurdles to overcome in our struggle to achieve a desirable body weight. Among them are the following:

1. AMERICANS LOVE FAD DIETS.

We Americans are always looking for a quick fix. There's a long history of attaching ourselves to fad diets, dating back to the Vinegar Diet in 1820. Since then, we've tried everything, from the oat bran craze to low-fat/high-protein to gluten-free diets. Unfortunately, none of these diets allows us to sustain weight loss.

Dieting is also an expensive habit. Americans spend about $40 billion annually on diet programs, meals, supplements and fads. The reality is that *each encounter with a fad diet has been proven to inhibit or delay weight loss, rather than initiate and sustain it.*

2. THE FOOD INDUSTRY PUTS PROFITS FIRST, OUR HEALTH SECOND.

For almost 20 years, I was one of the first nutrition consultants for a supermarket chain—and it didn't take long for me to become a disenchanted dietitian. I observed how food companies manipulate customers into buying foods with "empty" calories (those with no nutritional value). Because grocers earn more money selling potato chips, sodas and hot dogs than they do fresh fruits and vegetables, these products get priority placement on supermarket shelves.

3. ADVERTISERS FILL US WITH FALSE HOPES.

The American advertising industry is notorious for manipulating the public into buying goods that are not necessarily in their best interests. Wherever we look are promises of hope in a can, bottle or package. Check the shelves: There are diet pills, diet drinks, expensive weight-loss machines and other contraptions that ultimately end up in the garbage or in a yard sale. When a new medical study comes out, new products are sure to follow, even if the study is insignificant and unconfirmed.

This also applies to confusing information on food choices (studies that say "avoid eggs," followed soon after by studies that advise us to "eat more eggs"). Madison Avenue contributes to our confusion when we're trying to follow a healthy lifestyle, but we can change that.

4. AMERICANS TRUST THEIR DOCTORS, BUT...

Most physicians have good intentions, but their training is focused on prescribing medications, such as appetite suppressants and pills to lower cholesterol or control blood sugars. While medications and pills may provide relief, they can also create other problems within the body. For example, it's known that statins (popular cholesterol-lowering medications) cause muscle fatigue and are possible culprits in increasing the risks of diabetes and depression.

When it comes to nutrition, a registered dietitian is your best go-to expert about weight issues and diet. Once your MD has ruled out any possible illness, a dietitian will suggest the right nutritional options for you personally, with the goal to achieve safe, long-term weight loss.

Best of all, a healthy diet can often get people off medications for hypertension, diabetes and high cholesterol!

5

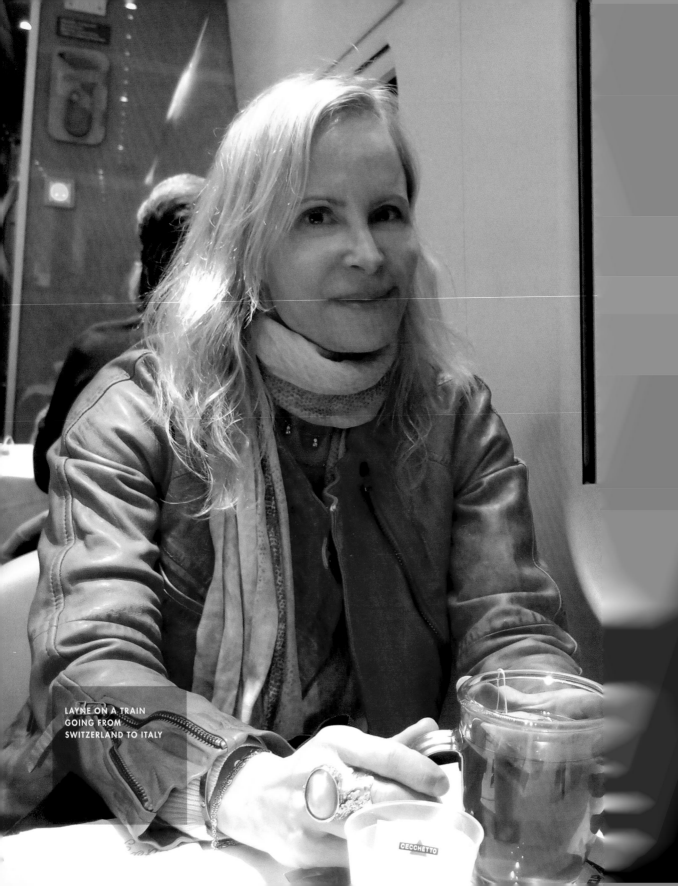

LAYNE ON A TRAIN
GOING FROM
SWITZERLAND TO ITALY

MY LIFELONG SEARCH FOR THE HEALTHIEST DIET

admit it—I have always loved food! When I was a child, I couldn't wait for Saturday morning to make my own Big American Breakfast. Everything came out of the fridge that could possibly go into my omelet: diced ham, chopped onion and slices of American cheese. I would experiment with seasonings, sometimes salt and pepper, and other times lots of sugar! Food was my life.

My world came crashing down around me when I was diagnosed with dangerously high cholesterol at the age of nine. I learned that it could be controlled through changes in diet, so I had to say goodbye to my favorite breakfasts of overstuffed omelets, pancakes with bacon and cream cheese-slathered bagels. I also had to put aside—permanently—my regular lunch sandwich of piled-high ham and cheese on rye with lots of mayo. Dinners, which usually featured a different cut of beef every night, had to be replaced with healthier options.

I dove right in, switching from butter to margarine, (which I later realized was no better), and giving up my adored Twinkies and Devil Dogs. Then, I replaced meats with legumes, poultry and fish, and discovered tofu, lentils and brown rice. I learned to perfect the art of making egg-white omelets. I even taught local chefs how to make healthier egg salad by cutting back on the yolks.

By the time I was in high school, I was writing weekly articles for the local newspaper titled, "You Are What You Eat." I set a goal to attend the best university to study nutrition and biochemistry and was accepted to Cornell. Then I went on to graduate school at New York University and received a medical nutrition research fellowship at Albert Einstein College of Medicine.

I worked in almost every field of food and nutrition, eager to learn everything I could. I became a Registered Dietitian-Nutritionist and, in time, was a recognized expert in the field of nutrition. (Just a note: Doctors, coaches and counselors who call themselves "diet experts" often have no comprehensive training in nutrition; so if you're seeking dietary advice, be sure they have an RD after their names.)

As I found answers to my own diet questions, I felt a powerful calling to help others struggling with their personal food dilemmas. In the 1980s I opened "Nutrition Learning Centers," which combined cooking classes, a health food store and nutrition counseling.

7

Good Morning America invited me on air as a nutrition expert at the age of 27 to share the success stories of my young clients who were enrolled in my Shape-Down Program.

I successfully counseled over 1,000 clients, wrote weekly articles in two newspapers, appeared regularly on News 12, and managed a staff of registered dietitians. When a grocery chain contacted me, seeking advice on how to help consumers who were looking for nutrition information, I realized that I could reach an even broader audience.

For 20 years, I worked in the supermarket industry as a consulting nutritionist and director of nutrition, but I began to become concerned about packaging, marketing and shelf-life issues. My days were filled convincing our buyers to work with local farmers, so our customers could enjoy the freshest fruits and vegetables with excellent nutritional value. However, the bottom line didn't always work out.

There were also weekly deadlines for newsletters, circular ads (where I had to be sure I didn't offend the junk food purveyors), recipes and web copy to write, while juggling my duties to explain why consumers should *not* follow the current fad diet.

For years, as a nutritionist and dietitian, I continued to search for a way to help others overcome the temptation to eat foods that led to obesity, and to avoid all the health problems—and healthcare costs—overeating brings.

I found out that trying to break the grip of fattening fast foods was no easy job! While a tsunami of diet books promised results, no specific program was successful over the long term. Disappointed dieters would quickly gain back the weight they lost—and then some—shortly after they fell off the diet wagon.

Clearly, we were having a tough time taking control of our diets and changing our eating habits. When my husband received a job offer in Geneva, Switzerland, I jumped at the chance to learn how Europeans lived healthier and longer lives while enjoying food.

To my surprise and delight, it was during my two years as an expatriate in Europe that I realized that the solution to our obesity and health crises could be found in the cuisines and lifestyles of three European countries—Switzerland, Italy and France. These three countries have amazing health statistics—with the best health scores in Europe!

They also have the longest life expectancies (Switzerland is #2 in the world) and some of the lowest rates of heart disease, diabetes and obesity in Europe. Yet their people continue to enjoy the foods we all long for, including pasta, cheese, bread, chocolate and wine.

I quickly realized that these countries would be excellent role models for us all, including our children and grandchildren, thanks to their superior diets and lifestyles.

Part One of this book explains why the diets of Switzerland, Italy and France are so impressive, and how they go *Beyond the* traditional *Mediterranean Diet!*

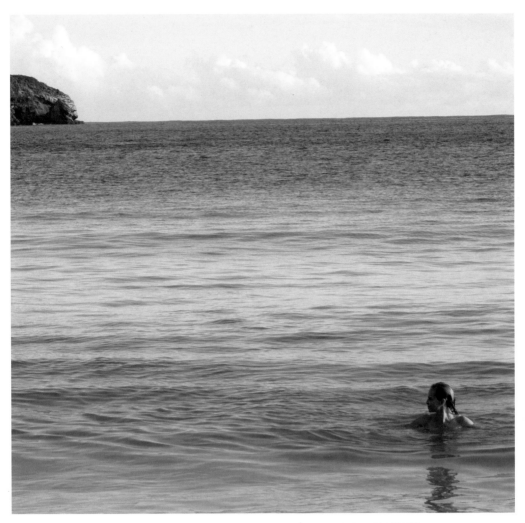

LAYNE IN THE CARIBBEAN SEA, SAINT BARTHÉLEMY, FRENCH WEST INDIES

Part Two introduces the tools you'll need to incorporate this knowledge into your daily life: the "Super-Healthy Plate;" six easy steps to adopting the European-style diet; helpful food-shopping tips; and a guide to ordering with confidence when dining out.

Part Three offers easy, delicious, low-fat recipes for breakfast, lunch, dinner, snacks and desserts, along with nutritional analysis. The recipes are simple, yet creative, using natural ingredients with a European twist. And there are a wide variety of vegetarian and gluten-free recipes mixed in. The Appendix also provides a wealth of information and resources.

Now, let's explore how going *Beyond the Mediterranean Diet* can change your life and add years to it—and to those of the people you love most.

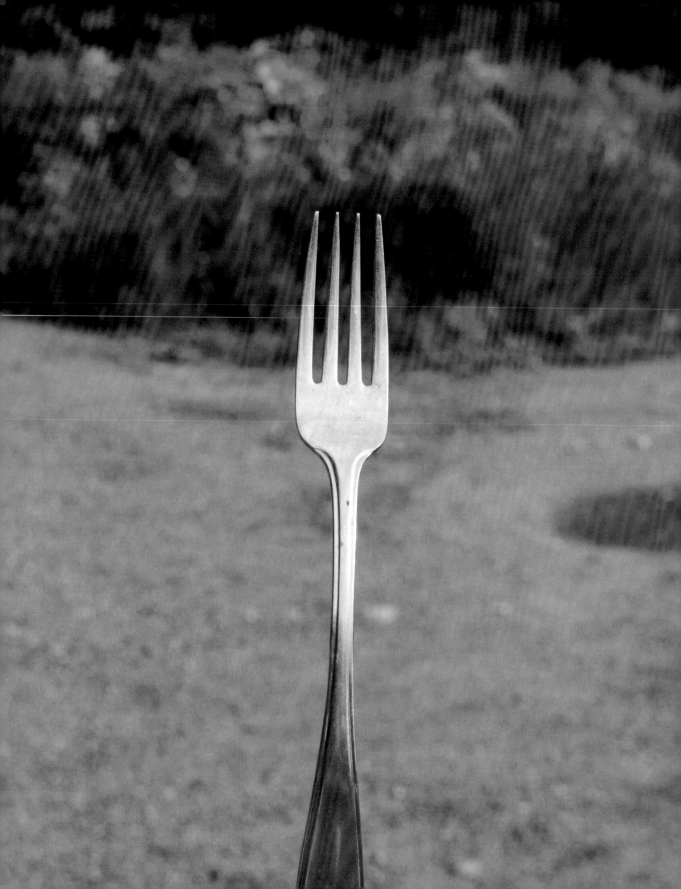

Part One

A FORK IN THE ROAD—AND A REVELATION!

11

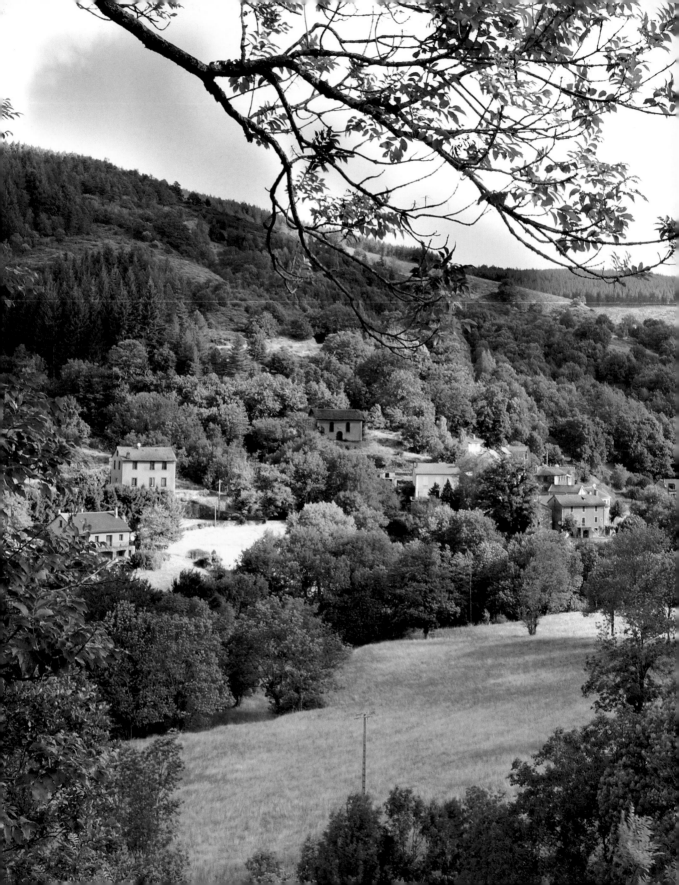

Chapter 1

DISCOVERING EUROPE'S THREE HEALTHIEST COUNTRIES

13

SMALL TOWN IN
THE FOOTHILLS OF
THE FRENCH ALPS

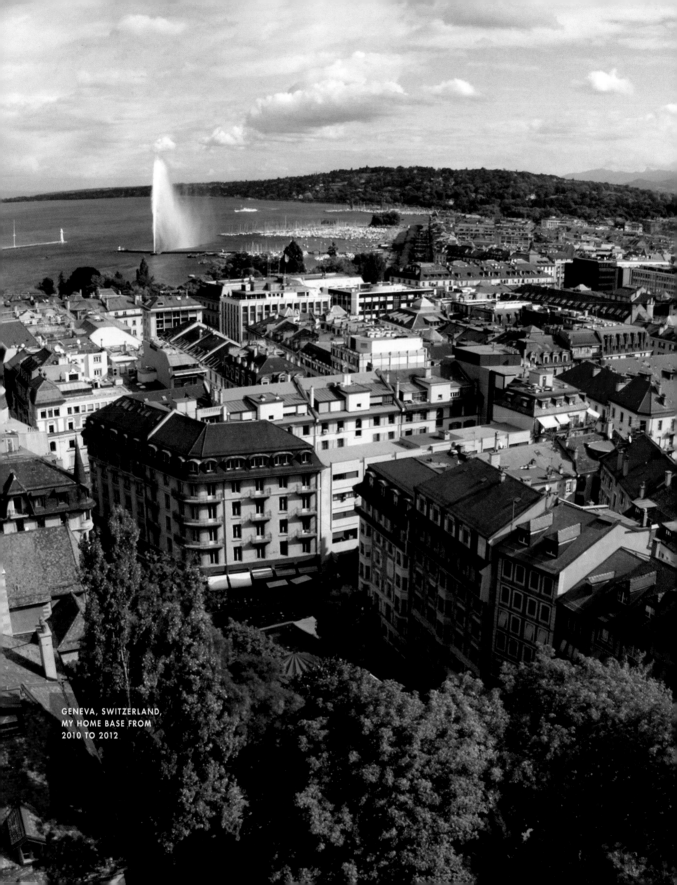

GENEVA, SWITZERLAND,
MY HOME BASE FROM
2010 TO 2012

When my husband, Michael, received a job offer from a global engineering firm to move to Switzerland, I saw it as an opportunity to experience the food culture and explore the dietary habits of Europe firsthand! And the unexpected happened: I found the answer I had been looking for, right there in front of me on a Swiss International Airlines meal tray (we were able to fly business class) as I flew across the ocean to my new life abroad.

That flight was, to put it mildly, a real eye-opener. Unlike the disappointing airline meals in our country, I found before me a dish of *tagliatelle* with fresh vegetables and roasted chestnuts. What a revelation—I never expected to find heaven on a plate in an airplane! I still recall the vibrant array of fragrances and flavors that were tantalizing my taste buds.

Following this delicious appetizer, I was offered a choice of smoked duck breast with a pear and celery salad, beef filet with an alpine herb crust, or chicken with pumpkin risotto. I thought to myself, "If this is just airplane food, what can I expect when I visit a European restaurant?"

Living abroad turned into a life-changing adventure. It restored my passion for food—a passion that had begun to fade over the years. Food tasted good again, thanks to the fresh ingredients in every dish. European food culture is rich with tradition and ingenuity. I saw families from all economic backgrounds visiting the farmers markets in cities and villages every week, seeking high-quality, fresh foods for their families. They learned which farmers cared most about how they grew and raised their food. They cared not only for the health of their families, but also for the well-being of the land.

For the next two years, I immersed myself in European culture so I could truly understand diets, habits and lifestyles. I visited markets, studying the ingredients, communities and cooking of a wide range of countries. I also got to know the chefs, locals and farmers. Everywhere I went, I made notes, tasting and eating fresh foods (and staying slender)! I was re-energized and inspired in my new environment and rediscovered the passion for food from my youth.

I came to realize that a cluster of countries had the best health statistics in Europe. Out of 17 of the most affluent countries in the world, Switzerland, Italy and France rank in the top five for life span. Sadly, the United States ranks last.

According to a recent National Research Council's comparison of longevity for the world's 17 most affluent countries, Switzerland ranks #2, Italy ranks #4 and France ranks #5. (Japan ranks #1.) People in these three countries have learned to walk the line between staying healthy and enjoying their beloved foods. They are aware of the obesity epidemic and avoid falling into the traps that are detrimental to health: oversized portions, processed foods and fad diets.

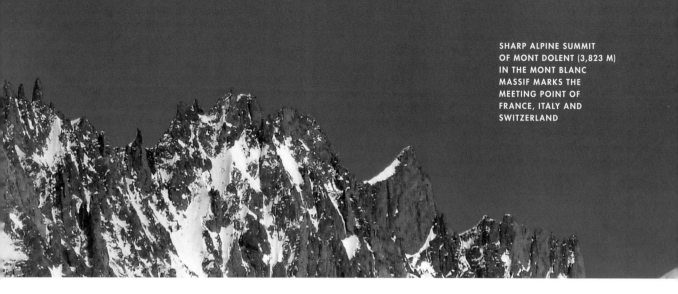

You may read that Europeans are expanding their waistlines, but keep in mind that while 68 percent of Americans are overweight or obese (Journal of the American Medical Association, 2010) according to the Organization for Economic Co-operation and Development, the obesity rate in Switzerland, Italy and France is around one-quarter of that in the U.S.! That's because on average, Americans consume about 4,000 calories a day—more than anyone else in the world!

The following health statistics regarding Switzerland, Italy, France and the U.S. are compiled from the World Health Organization, Eurostat and the Centers for Disease Control and Prevention (CDC).

Switzerland boasts one of the lowest obesity rates in Europe, averaging 8 percent (2007). This country also has the second highest life expectancy rate of industrialized countries (age 82) and a coronary heart disease death rate of 52.2 per 100,000 persons (2011). The death rate from diabetes is 8.2 per 100,000 persons (2011).

Surprisingly, considering all the pizza and pasta consumed by Italians, their obesity rate is only about 9.8 percent (2005). In Italy, the death rate from coronary heart disease is a modest 51.7 per 100,000 persons (2011). The death rate from diabetes is 12.4 per 100,000 persons (2011).

France boggles the mind with the lowest rate of coronary heart disease deaths in the European Union at 29.2 per 100,000 persons (2011). The death rate from diabetes is also at a low 8.0 per 100,000 persons (2011). Furthermore, obesity in France is an impressive 16.9 percent (2007).

In contrast, the United States has the highest rate of obesity in the world at a whopping 35.7 percent (2009 to 2010). Coronary heart disease death rate remains high at a staggering 80.5 per 100,000 persons (2011). The death rate from diabetes is also high at 15.2 per 100,000 persons (2011). According to the American Diabetes Association the total cost of diabetes was $245 billion in 2012. According to the American Heart

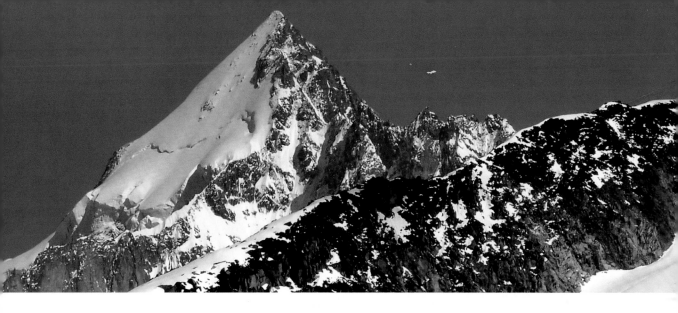

Association, costs associated with heart disease will reach $818.1 billion a year by 2030. The future of the U.S. health economy looks bleak.

As I dug deeper into these statistics, I learned that the people of Switzerland, Italy and France consume less sugar, less fruit juice and fewer soft drinks than those in the U.S. They also snack less, spend less time eating and more time socializing at meals. They eat smaller breakfasts, larger lunches and smaller dinners.

Portion sizes alone are an eye-opener, with an emphasis on quality versus quantity. Bottles of soda are 6 ounces, versus the 20- to 64-ounce supersizes here in the United States. Muffins, bagels and doughnuts are easily five times larger in the U.S. than in Europe. And Europeans don't even snack on them. They sell them to the tourists!

Europeans don't obsess about counting calories, carbs and fat grams; instead, they rely on their instincts, almost as if their bodies have a built-in counter! Europeans follow healthy habits, routines, and attitudes when it comes to food. Reading food labels on packaged food is less effective than actually touching, smelling and tasting fresh food.

Europeans know that good food costs more, and they willingly spend more than 10 percent of their incomes on food. In comparison, France spends 14 percent, and Americans spend 6 percent of their household expenditures on food. In fact, according to the Bill & Melinda Gates Foundation, Americans spend a smaller percentage of their income on food than people in any other country in the world!

For all the above reasons, people in this cluster of European countries—Switzerland, Italy and France—are truly the best role models for health-conscious people to follow, wherever they live.

What I had been searching for in the United States was now right before my eyes. I knew exactly what I needed to do to improve the health statistics and fight the obesity epidemic both at home and abroad.

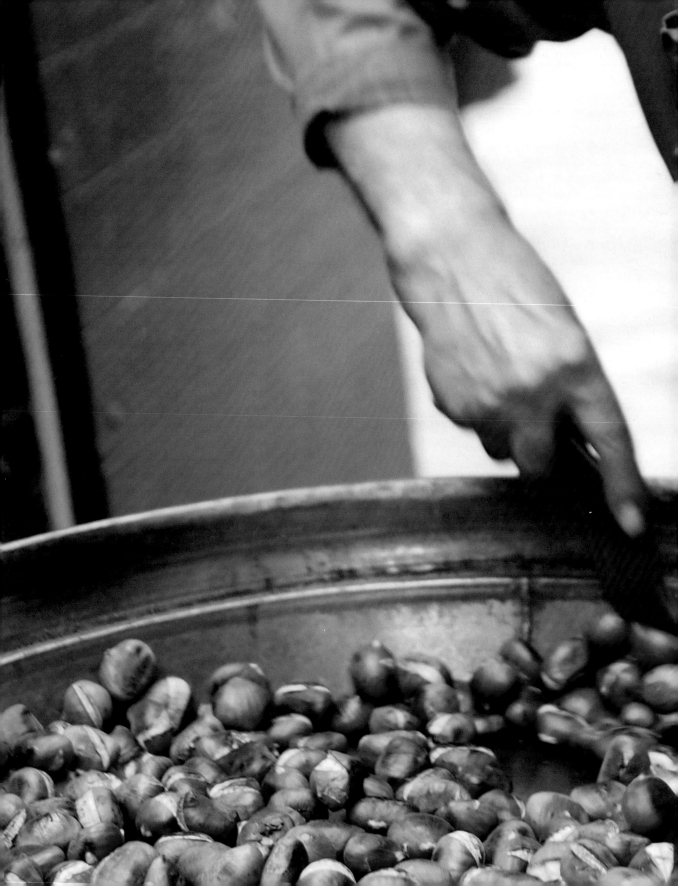

Chapter 2

THE SECRETS OF THE SWISS DIET

FAVORITE AFTERNOON
SNACK OF ROASTED
CHESTNUTS AT A HUT ON
RUE DE RIVE, GENEVA,
SWITZERLAND

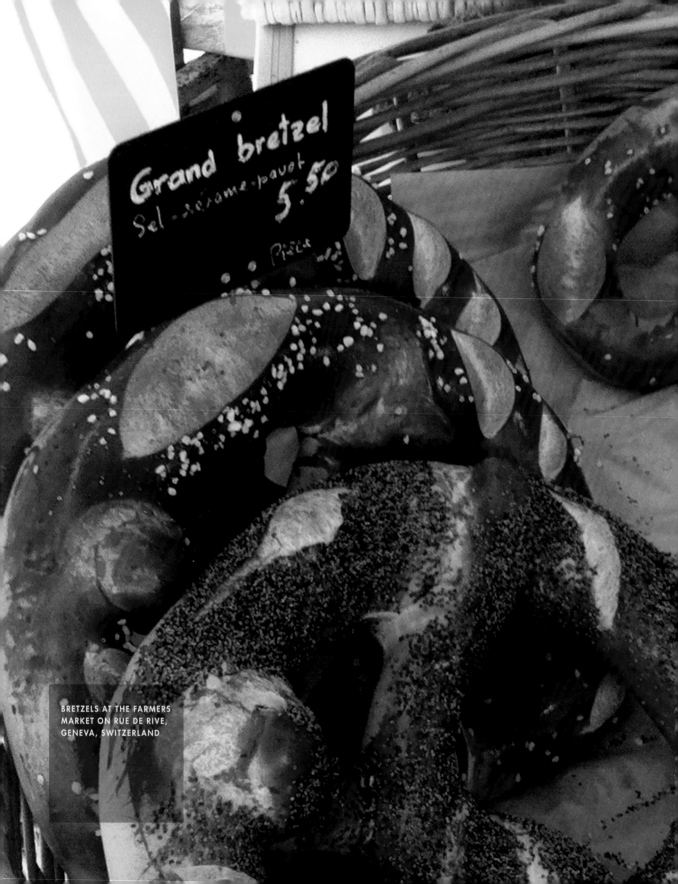

Grand bretzel
Sel - sesame - pavot
5.50
Pièce

BRETZELS AT THE FARMERS
MARKET ON RUE DE RIVE,
GENEVA, SWITZERLAND

How is it possible for a country famed for its chocolates and cheeses to have the lowest obesity rate in Europe? Incredibly, only eight percent of the Swiss are obese, compared with over 30 percent of Americans. Is the secret "good genes" or a special ingredient in their water that keeps the Swiss so slim?

Actually, the answer lies in the Swiss formula for a fit and wholesome lifestyle. It explains the country's ranking as number one in Europe and second in the world for the longest life span out of 17 of the most affluent nations.

Switzerland's enforcement of strict agricultural trade policies, its concern for animal welfare and its prohibitions on industrialized farming, pave the way to satisfy its citizens' hearty appetite for wholesome food. The Swiss agricultural industry provides about 60 percent of the nation's food needs, with over two-thirds of the industry focusing on milk, meat, poultry and eggs. The other one-third specializes in fruits, vegetables and wines.

Organic farming is a way of life, and 11 percent of farms are organic; in comparison, in the U.S. only about two percent of the food supply is grown organically. I've been told that no other European country besides Denmark buys as much organic food as the Swiss. The Swiss don't mind spending a little more money as an investment in their health.

Besides their love of organic food, the Swiss also support the environment and appreciate that organic farming is better for the land as well as for their health.

21

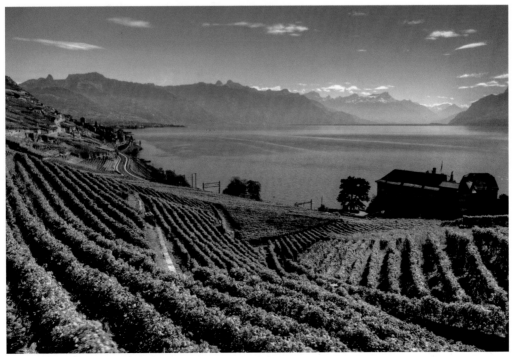

TERRACED VINEYARDS FACING THE SHORES OF LAKE GENEVA—ALSO KNOWN AS LAKE LÉMAN, SWITZERLAND

Although Switzerland is known worldwide for precision instruments, pharmaceutical products and high-valued currency, locals are enamored with its food and farming. With so many farmers markets in the cities and towns, it's obvious that the Swiss truly value seasonal fruits and vegetables, artisan breads and such national favorites (even if high in fat and calories) as fine chocolates, world-renowned cheeses (like Gruyère and Emmental) and biodynamic wines.

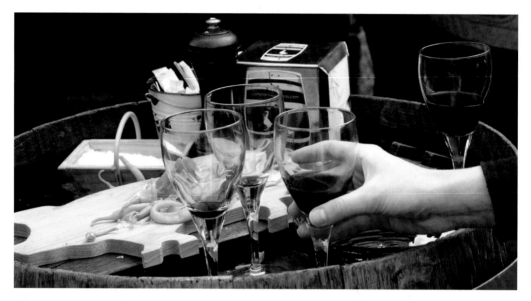

SATURDAY AFTERNOON SCENE NEAR A FARMERS MARKET IN SWITZERLAND

Biodynamic wineries actually exceed the standards of certified organic farming. Here, the vineyard's natural resources are used to cultivate the highest quality grapes without pesticides, fungicides, herbicides, synthetic fertilizers, growth stimulants or genetically modified organisms (GMOs). (See Appendix for further information about biodynamic, organic and sustainable wines.)

In fact, the Swiss love their wines so much, very few are exported. And they would never give up their cherished chocolates to conform to a diet that eliminated them.

There is one dish that unites this tiny multi-cultural country (it's smaller than West Virginia)—fondue, which means "melted" in French. Thanks to promotions by the Swiss Cheese Union, fondue has been the national dish since the 1930s.

Traditional fondue is a combination of melted Gruyère and Emmental cheese and wine, kept warm in a communal pot and served with chunks of crusty bread. You'll love this experience only if you love the aroma of warm cheese. The typical serving size is about one-half cup, which amounts to 250 calories and 16 grams of fat. It's the perfect snack after a long day of skiing! The Swiss enjoy it with a glass of white wine—never red, and never beer.

Raclette is the other national "cheesy" dish occasionally eaten by locals. I've seen *raclette* served as street food in Zurich. The name is derived from the French word *racler,* meaning "to scrape." The Swiss love to heat a large wedge of *raclette* cheese under a broiler, heating element or open flame until the surface is melted and gooey; then, the cheese is scraped onto a warm plate. *Raclette* is often served with fingerling potatoes, pickled onions and mini pickles, or gherkins. One ounce of *raclette* (about the size of a one-inch cube) is 100 calories and eight grams of fat.

A serving size can be four ounces or more, so this is *not* a heart-healthy dish. However, it's still better than a fast food burger composed of an unknown mixture of meat (and meat by-products), with a whopping 630 calories and 35 grams of fat.

With all this talk about eating cheese, take note that the Swiss produce mostly cow's-milk cheese. As with everything else they produce, wholesomeness is a priority, and cheese is no exception. Swiss cows eat grass in summer and hay in winter; they are not fed silage—stored and fermented grass crops. Silage often produces gas that can cause serious respiratory distress for farm workers and sometimes detrimental bacteria that can cause digestive problems for cows.

23

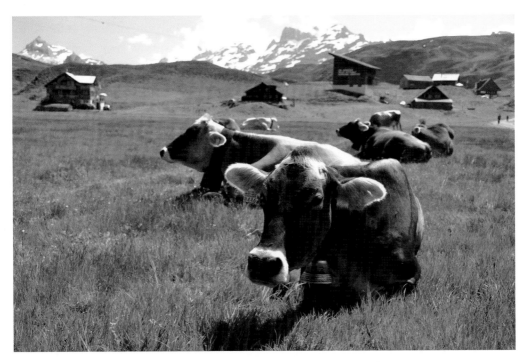

COWS IN AN ALPINE MEADOW IN SWITZERLAND

Most cheese is made with unpasteurized milk in small batches and often in the mountains where the cows graze. This is far different than in the U.S., where cheese aged less than 60 days must be made with pasteurized milk. Only cheese aged more than 60 days can be made with "raw" or unpasteurized milk. Pasteurization is a heating process, which slows spoilage by decreasing the bacterial count. Proponents of raw milk argue that if cows are fed and handled hygienically, harmful bacteria would not propagate in the milk. Heating milk (pasteurization) destroys some of the nutrients and probiotics (beneficial bacteria). In the U.S., federal law prohibits selling raw milk from state to state, but allows states to regulate its sale within their borders. In Europe, raw milk is legal but well regulated to ensure high health standards.

Cheese is an excellent source of protein and calcium; however, some varieties can be high in sodium, so choose those under 200 milligrams of sodium per serving. If you are on a sodium-restricted diet, go even lower. Fresh cheeses like ricotta cheese and farmer cheese are lowest in sodium. Because the U.S. agricultural industry supports factory farming, it's best to choose cheese that's organic or bovine growth hormone-free (rBGH-free) and lower in fat, like Jarlsberg Lite imported from Norway. Bovine growth hormone is banned in Europe. If a product is labeled organic it does not contain added hormones.

The Swiss produce and eat many varieties of fresh and aged cheeses, but they don't eat processed cheese, like American cheese. They prefer small quantities of high-quality cheese and are content without the addition of meat in their sandwiches. Maintaining a balanced diet is always their objective when selecting food for themselves and their families. I found this attention to healthful eating an admirable aspect of the Swiss identity.

As chocolate lovers are probably aware, many of the world's classic favorites are Swiss, such as Toblerone, Lindt, Ovaltine and Nestlé.

In 1819, F-L. Cailler opened the first Swiss chocolate factory. In 1866, Henri Nestlé opened the first Swiss condensed-milk factory. Together, they combined chocolate with condensed milk and invented milk chocolate! Nestlé later bought the Cailler Chocolate Company, and today Nestlé is the world's largest food company.

Another popular Swiss food invention is *muesli*, a wholesome breakfast cereal composed of uncooked oats, fruit and nuts. A Swiss physician named Maximilian Bircher-Benner developed it around 1900. Today, the term *muesli* is found on cereal boxes around the world. And just for you, I've created a healthy, delicious recipe for *muesli* in Part Three—enjoy!

Besides food production, Swiss authorities also regulate operating hours of businesses and shops. Stores (and often restaurants) are closed on Sundays. If the Swiss run out of milk, bread or have no food at home, they'll have to stop at the train station or a gas stop along the highway. The food in these places is of the same quality as that in the supermarket, as the same companies operate both. By closing stores on Sunday, the Swiss actually promote a higher quality of life and remove the temptation to leave one's family to go shopping.

In addition to benefiting from a variety of local foods, the Swiss enjoy scenic alpine and lake settings—a perfect backdrop for an outdoor lifestyle of skiing, biking, boating, hiking, etc. Weekends are centered on outdoor activities with family and friends. Evenings are for strolling, even during cold winter months. We can learn a lot from the Swiss about how to balance their love of wholesome food while staying physically active.

LAYNE'S SWISS FAVORITES

Switzerland comprises three distinct cultural regions: Swiss French, Swiss German and Swiss Italian, each with its own language and food. For two years I lived in the Swiss French city of Geneva, adjacent to a beautiful lake and surrounded by mountains. Geneva is the largest French-speaking city in Switzerland, bordered mostly by France.

Geneva was the perfect base for me to research this book. Its central location provided easy access to other countries where I could effortlessly learn to live and eat like a European. And it became easy to reset my palate and begin to experience the fresh, delicious food offered in this health-conscious country.

As a "mostly" vegetarian, I did a lot of cooking at home while living in Switzerland. While the vegan, raw food and vegetarian movements are slowly taking hold, it is still difficult to find a café or restaurant that caters to this need. The Swiss typically favor Indian restaurants when they want to eat vegetarian food.

The downside is that most Indian foods, vegetarian or not, are high in fat, calories and sodium. Sauces and curries are typically made with heavy cream and ghee (clarified butter), and many types of bread are deep-fried.

The good news is that Swiss supermarkets offer a wide selection of vegan and vegetarian options. Besides the abundance of local and organic produce, there are many "prepared food" choices such as lightly seasoned tofu, herb tofu sausage, pumpkin gnocchi and whole grain spätzle. Lightly dressed salads include lentil, couscous, carrot and beet. Unlike

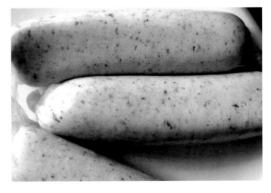

TOFU SAUSAGE FROM LA MAISON DU TOFU OF CAROUGE, SWITZERLAND

in the U.S., salads are not dripping with calorie-laden dressings or piled high with fried toppings.

While I was living in Geneva, my French girlfriend, Sophie, opened a cutting-edge (for Geneva) weekday café called "I Feel Bio." It has an exposed kitchen and cooking laboratory where recipes are developed for its detox program. The menu is changed daily based on what is available locally and organically.

A few of my favorites were: raw zucchini lasagna with cashew cheese, pressé de légumes (thin layers of sliced vegetables) au pesto (with pesto) and a delicious tarte aux fruits crue (fruit tart). Although the restaurant is not wholly vegetarian, the menu offers vegan, raw and vegetarian options daily.

In addition to imaginative dishes and desserts, Sophie offers an interesting assortment of daily teas, wines and homemade elixirs. She has access to the best collection

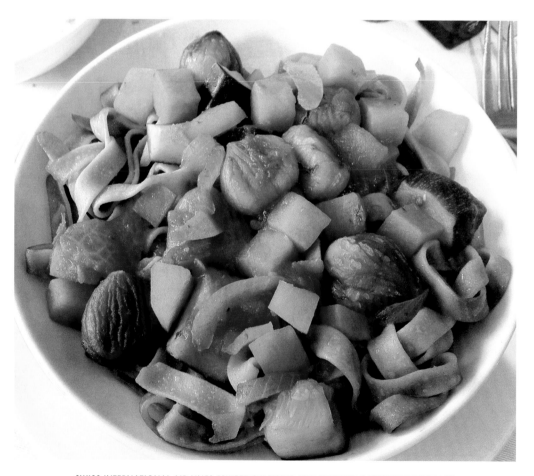

SWISS INTERNATIONAL AIR LINES "SWEET CHESTNUT AND PUMPKIN RATATOUILLE SPINACH TAGLIATELLE," CREATED BY HILTL VEGETARIAN RESTAURANT OF ZURICH, SWITZERLAND

of biodynamic wine in Geneva. Her café is quite atypical for Geneva, a city known for more traditional dining.

The oldest vegetarian restaurant in the world is Hiltl, which continues to operate in the Swiss German city of Zurich. It opened in 1898, but today the restaurant is as vibrant as ever under the fourth-generation direction of Rolf Hiltl. The owner was kind enough to give me a tour of both Hiltl and a newer vegetarian venture called "tibits."

Today, Swiss, the national airline, features a Hiltl menu on all intercontinental flights departing from Switzerland. My favorite dish was the "Sweet Chestnut and Pumpkin Ratatouille Spinach Tagliatelle" which was deliciously light and satisfying. I found the Swiss Germans more inclined to eat vegetarian, perhaps as a contrast to the more traditional, "rich" German food.

A favorite Swiss food spot is at the center of Europe's alpine mountain range, the Swiss Alps, offering numerous culinary treasures. It is here that French, Italian and Swiss foods merge on mountaintops. Swiss families often focus their ski trips around food as well as snow conditions. On the slopes, you can always count on hearty, traditional fare. Tarts, open pastries, salads and quiches are commonly served in the French areas, while pizza, pasta and minestrone soup are staples in the Italian sections. Wherever you are, be sure to drink a Swiss hot chocolate!

The high-fat foods of the alpine region support the finding that active people in cold climates eat higher calorie foods. This does not equate to fried, processed and often nutritionally devoid foods in our "fast food nation." Even though American ski resorts were inspired by Swiss ski villages, our resorts serve foil-wrapped burgers on a plastic tray!

27

SWISS DIETARY GUIDELINES

Switzerland's Federal Office of Public Health uses the Swiss Food Pyramid developed by the Swiss Society for Nutrition. It's very different from our American one, which ignores water and places grains before fruits and vegetables. (See Appendix for 2005 USDA Food Pyramid.) The Swiss Pyramid recommends:

1. The majority of dietary protein from milk and dairy, three portions per day.
2. One (three- to four-ounce) portion of protein per day: either meat, fish, eggs, tofu or other protein.
3. At least three portions of vegetables and two portions of different-colored fruit per day.

4. Three portions of whole grains, potatoes and pulses (beans and lentils) per day.
5. Oils, nuts and other fats daily, in moderation.
6. One to two liters (about four to eight cups) of unsweetened beverages (preferably water) per day.
7. Sweet/salty snacks and sweetened/alcoholic drinks in moderation for pleasure (as opposed to nutrition).

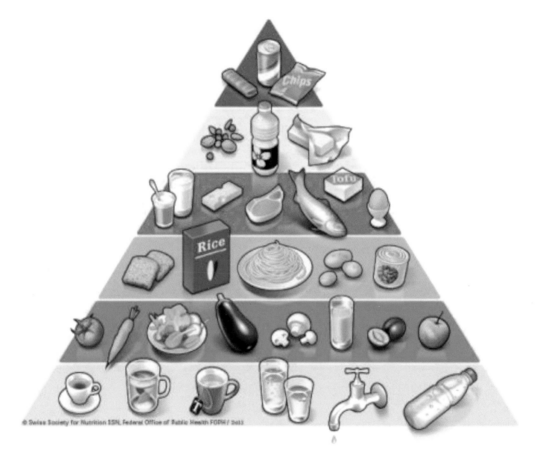

THE SWISS FOOD PYRAMID

I was fascinated to learn that the Swiss do not follow America's trend of eating less fat. Instead, the Swiss recommend 30 to 40 percent of daily calories from fat, while the American Heart Association recommends 30 percent. The Swiss guidelines recommend consuming two to three tablespoons of oils, one portion of unsalted nuts or seeds, and up to one tablespoon of butter, margarine or cream per day.

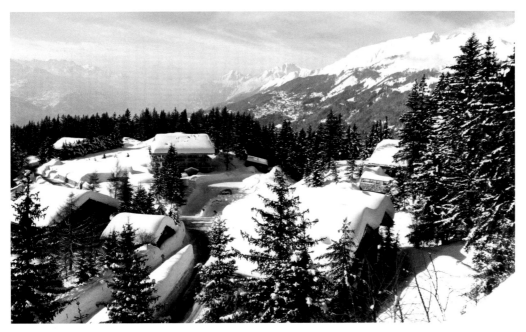

OUTDOOR SCENE AT HOTEL LeCRANS IN CRANS-MONTANA, SWITZERLAND

Do keep in mind that Switzerland, with its alpine climate, is one of the coldest central European countries. People in colder climates traditionally eat heavier foods. Since shivering burns calories, cold weather may boost your caloric burn, too. Just don't use it as an excuse to go overboard!

Because the Swiss are far more active and sports-oriented than other countries, including the U.S., try not to follow the Swiss' fat intake recommendations. For instance, on most summer weekends, Swiss families will go swimming or hiking; in winter, they will switch to skiing in the powdery snow of the Alps. I suggest that countries with a less active lifestyle follow the American Heart Association's recommendation of no more than 30 percent (in a less active lifestyle, 20 to 25 percent is an even better goal) of daily calories from fat.

As to indulging in sweets, the Swiss believe that a little indulgence is fine. They consume sweets, salty snacks and alcohol in moderation, such as a small square of chocolate with tea mid-morning or a handful of salted almonds midday. A 2013 report says Swiss alcohol consumption is declining, and consumers are focusing more on quality than quantity. Migros, Switzerland's largest supermarket chain—considered a Swiss institution since 1925—does not sell alcohol or tobacco products.

The Swiss present a balanced approach to indulging without overdoing it. Compare this to the United States' latest version of a food guide, "MyPlate," which fails to limit quantities of sweets, salty snacks and alcohol—all of which contribute to our obesity epidemic! (See Appendix for USDA 2011 MyPlate.)

The Swiss do not judge foods as "good" or "bad;" instead, they emphasize the importance of a varied diet that includes locally produced, non-factory farmed foods— from potatoes and red meat to omelets and desserts.

The only "must" is the daily intake of fluids, preferably water. The Swiss recommend drinking one to two liters (1.06 to 2.12 quarts) per day. I often saw locals walking around with recyclable bottles filled with clear tap water. As to bottled water, this appears only when one is in the mood for sparkling or flat mineral water at a café or restaurant.

The Swiss understand that they must be active to be able to maintain a healthy body weight. They aim for at least 30 minutes of outdoor activity daily, balanced with sufficient relaxation.

Numerous studies have demonstrated the advantages of outdoor sports over indoor ones, so this is not surprising. If you are unable to be outdoors, suffer from milk allergies, or adhere to strict vegan diets, you may be at risk for vitamin D deficiency. A mere fifteen minutes of sunshine daily will help your body manufacture this nutrient, which promotes calcium absorption to protect you against osteoporosis. It also has a role in immune function and reduces inflammation.

30

Obese people often have low blood levels of vitamin D.

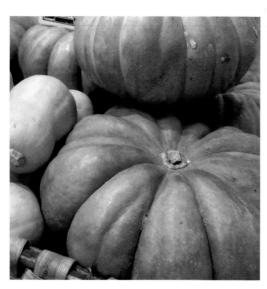

PUMPKINS AT A FRENCH MARKET

Scientists suggest that vitamin D gets diluted as it moves through the body, and shows up as a deficiency in overweight and obese individuals. As you add weight and volume to your body, your skin surface does not expand proportionately, and leads to insufficient vitamin D absorption.

I loved the outdoor lifestyle of the Swiss and often biked in the countryside on the outskirts of Geneva. One Saturday, I discovered the Fall Pumpkin Festival in Corsier, a municipality of Geneva. Corsier is also where the first Swiss chocolate factory was built. Food stands were bursting with pumpkin bread, paella, barrels of apples, jugs of cider and a myriad of pumpkins and gourds in every shape and size.

Unlike at American fairs and festivals, there were no hot dogs, burgers or funnel cakes. Instead, wholesome food from local suppliers was in abundance, to the delight of the entire town and its visitors.

In summary, our lesson from the Swiss centers on the importance of eating a diet rich in wholesome (unprocessed) foods. The active Swiss lifestyle keeps appetites high and bodies slender. Now, let's explore more about Switzerland's outstanding dietary habits. This will help you understand how they preserve a high quality of life, support the integrity of local food producers, and can satisfy the palates of a multi-cultural population.

THE HEALTHY SWISS DIET

Organic or *"bio"* foods are commonly found everywhere, in supermarkets, farmers markets, train stations and gas station stops. Even conventionally produced foods in Switzerland contain fewer preservatives and additives compared to American foods, which often have artificial and natural additives to "boost" flavor.

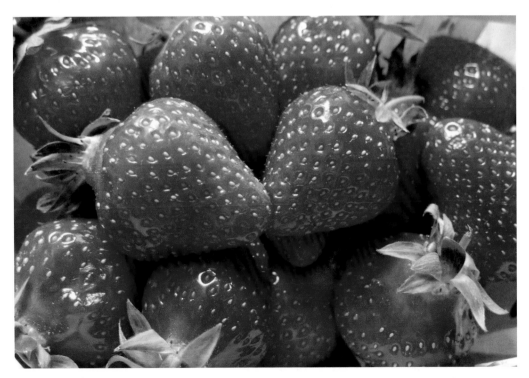

SUMMER STRAWBERRIES FROM THE FARMERS MARKET ON RUE DE RIVE IN GENEVA, SWITZERLAND

American food companies add these flavors to maintain a consistent taste experience so repeat customers won't complain that a product tastes different, depending on where and when they buy it. What we fail to acknowledge is that food is about the "moment" of taste, not the "aftertaste."

I learned from the Swiss that an imported strawberry in winter never tastes as good as a local strawberry in summer! A food's flavor depends on soil, season and locale. When you actually taste the subtle differences in food, you no longer feel compelled to eat under-ripe, cold-stored, chemically preserved, artificially flavored and often nutritionally devoid food. Instead you look forward to what each season offers and appreciate delicious and nutritious food. Even in smaller doses, you are fully satisfied!

Switzerland, where family farms still exist, grows almost everything that can withstand its cold climate. Nearly every home has a garden with fruit trees. Popular staples include potatoes, beans, carrots, chard, cauliflower and spinach. Fruits, depending upon the season, include apples, pears, grapes and, during summer, a variety of berries.

The Swiss enjoy meat (mostly lamb and beef) and poultry (mostly chicken and game hens; turkey is less popular). The quality is outstanding because of the way the animals are fed and raised. Cattle and sheep are grass-fed on open pastures rather than being force-fed (a corn-based diet) in a confined area. Grass-fed animals are leaner and produce meat higher in omega-3 fatty acids, compared to corn-fed animals that produce meat higher in omega-6 fatty acids. Omega-3 fatty acids have an anti-inflammatory effect on the body, while some omega-6 fatty acids cause inflammation. Grass-fed animals also produce more CLA (conjugated linoleic acid), which reduces inflammation and strengthens immunity.

Grass-fed animals are different from organically raised animals, which are born and raised on certified organic feed and do not take antibiotics or growth-promoting hormones. Organically raised animals are often fed corn before being slaughtered. While grass-fed animals are raised primarily on a diet of foraged grass, the pasture does not have to be free of pesticides, and animals are not restricted from antibiotics or hormones.

Thus, your ideal meat would be both organic *and* grass-fed. But if you cannot find this selection, either grass-fed or organic are good alternatives.

Most grass-fed meat in the U.S. is imported from Australia and New Zealand. Unlike the Swiss, we tend to consume corn-fed beef, which may explain why our rates of obesity and disease are higher. Because Americans mostly import grass-fed meat, it is more expensive, so many of us will not buy it. However, once the taste is acquired, grass-fed meat is more satisfying, and smaller portions are enough to please every meat-eater.

It is rare to find a seafood restaurant in Switzerland, because Switzerland has lakes and is not surrounded by a sea. Supermarkets sell organic shrimp from Viet Nam and organic farm-raised salmon from Norway. Otherwise, local lake fish like bream, pike, perch and trout are common fare.

Seafood lovers visit the coastal regions of France, Italy and Spain when they crave the flavors of fish from the Mediterranean Sea. Switzerland, like the rest of Europe, is concerned about the decline in fish species. This has accelerated since houses appeared on the lake, river and sea banks, as well as the practices of over-fishing and increased pollution, just as in our country.

Dairy is the primary source of protein and a big part of the Swiss diet, with a smattering of low-fat varieties, but I could not find any fat-free alternatives. Just over the border in France, in the Carrefour's supermarket, I did find organic skim milk (*lait écrémé* means "skim milk" in French).

While fermented foods have recently become trendy in America, Switzerland has been producing them for ages. Fermentation occurs when sugars and carbohydrates in a food convert to something else. For example, juice is turned into wine, and grain is converted to beer. In addition to wine and beer, there are cultured milk products like yogurt and some cheeses.

Other fermented foods include sauerkraut, pickles, vinegar, cider and sourdough bread. In addition to enhancing flavors, fermentation prolongs shelf life. Fermented foods maintain the good bacteria in our intestines and can aid digestion. If you are lactose intolerant, you can usually tolerate cultured milk like yogurt or kefir, because the milk-sugar (lactase) is broken down, making it more digestible.

Some health experts endorse lactic-acid fermented foods, such as pickles and sauerkraut, as being especially rich in enzyme activity. This may help us better absorb the nutrients in our foods.

FOOD SHOPPING, SWISS-STYLE

Groceries are reasonably priced, but eating out in Switzerland is very expensive. Therefore, food shopping is an important part of Swiss life. Two companies, Coop and Migros, operate most of the food markets in Switzerland. Shoppers expand their range of foods by shopping at farmers markets, organic stores and specialty shops. It is common for department stores to have food markets on the lower level and gourmet cafeterias on the upper level. Locals and business people crowd these stores during lunchtime.

Coop and Migros offer extensive private-label organic and budget lines of foods, using mostly local ingredients. Both companies recognize that a high consumption

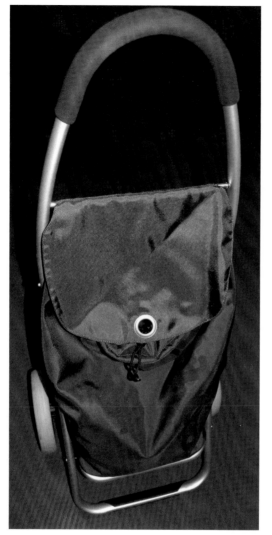

MY EUROPEAN SHOPPING CART

of saturated fats and trans-fatty acids is linked to heart disease. Therefore, as in the U.S., there is a trend to replace these fats with polyunsaturated vegetable oils in the small numbers of packaged foods they produce.

Switzerland is home to the Max-Havelaar Foundation, a member of Fairtrade International and an independent certifier that issues The Fairtrade trademark. This identifies products that follow an international standard for fair trade. Thanks to fair trade, the living standards and working conditions of small farmers in disadvantaged regions are improved.

Small-scale natural food markets exist and offer a variety of special dietary foods, but none can match the scale of America's Whole Foods or Trader Joe's markets. However, as a source of local, natural and organic foods, Switzerland's conventional supermarkets, farmers markets and natural food markets are more than sufficient for most needs.

In Switzerland, low-fat (one percent) and reduced-fat (two percent) milk are sold in unrefrigerated, sterilized boxes. Americans do not like to buy milk in this type of packaging, as "fresh" milk is usually found in the refrigerated dairy case. Swiss supermarkets also carry a selection of unrefrigerated milk alternatives like rice, soy and oat milk. However, these tend to be overly sweet, are not enriched, and differ from what we are used to in America. Dairy cases are instead filled with whole milk, yogurt, cheese and prepared foods.

Small refrigerators (probably regulated by the Swiss government) are one reason that the Swiss shop at least twice weekly for food. Many even shop daily and plan meals based on what they find available in the market. It is popular, and a good source of exercise, to walk to the food market with a fashionable "shopping cart."

Supermarkets promote traditional fare depending upon the season and holiday. For Christmas, you will find spice cakes and cookies made with ground hazelnuts and almonds. During Easter, displays will be brimming with chocolate eggs, bunnies, bonnets and baskets. Many regional holidays are also celebrated with food, like the *Fête de l'Escalade,* a festival held in December, only in Geneva, to celebrate the defeat of a surprise attack by a French duke in 1602. Chocolate pots are sold to symbolize the pots of soup poured on the troops to prevent them from climbing *(l'escalade)* the walls of the city.

The Swiss appreciate and take advantage of wholesome, local and organic foods right at their fingertips. They would never give up a visit to the farmers market for a dollar-menu meal at McDonald's!

SPECIALTY FOODS, SWISS STYLE

Freshly baked breads are important to the Swiss and come in a wide variety of shapes, sizes and types, depending on which region of Switzerland you are in. There's French-style crusty bread, German-style dense rye, and Italian-style flat *focaccia.* Variety abounds with different types of grains, from ancient varieties such as *einkorn* (ancient wheat), to rye, corn and oat. Some are seeded, and others are sweet. Local bakeries pride themselves on unique, handmade breads, and feature traditions passed down from one generation of bakers to the next.

The pretzel that is now eaten worldwide was invented in Munich, Germany, in 1839. Outdoor pretzel *(bretzel)* stands are popular throughout Switzerland. They offer many different seeded varieties (including pumpkin) and are sliced horizontally to make bretzel sandwiches. A thin slice of ham with butter is popular. ·

One of my favorite Swiss supermarket breads is savory cornbread, bursting with rich whole cornmeal and lightly dusted with coarse corn flour. I love the yellow color, hearty texture and fresh corn aroma. In the fall, during pumpkin season, local pumpkin bread is a favorite. Also popular is German-style *quark* bread—moist, sour and hearty. (Quark is a sour fresh cheese.)

Supermarkets rarely carry pre-sliced loaves, instead offering freshly baked breads throughout the day. There are no "day olds" here! Compare this to our supermarket breads, which are primarily pre-sliced wheat (often with just a touch of whole-wheat) and white, made on conveyor belts and filled with preservatives and stabilizers to last a week or more on the shelf.

Magenbrot (or sweet pieces of bread) is a Swiss-German version of *biscotti,* glazed hard biscuits similar in taste to gingerbread, and sold mostly during the Christmas season. Like biscotti, it's thought to aid in digestion with its mixture of spices—nutmeg, cloves, cinnamon and star anise. My favorite authentic and regional version, created by spice merchants over 700 years ago, is from Basel. Called *Basler Leckerli*, it is available in the U.S. online.

Cardon Epineux Genevois, from the same plant family as the artichoke, is grown in the Plainpalais area of Geneva, known for its grassy plain, the neighborhood in which I

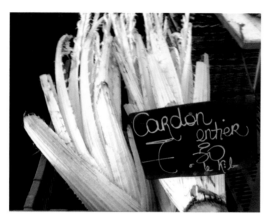

CARDON, A LOCAL VEGETABLE FROM PLAINPALAIS, AT A FARMERS MARKET IN GENEVA, SWITZERLAND

lived while in Switzerland. *Cardon* ("cardoon" in English) is a thorny, thistle-like, vagabond plant that spreads and grows rapidly. It is found throughout Geneva and eaten during the Christmas and New Year season. It's low calorie, high in fiber and brimming with nutrients like B-vitamins (a good amount of folic acid), vitamin C, calcium, iron, magnesium, potassium and lots of trace minerals, including selenium.

The vegetable is available in a jar or raw, and tastes like a cross between artichoke and Swiss chard. The flower buds can be eaten like an artichoke. The stems and stalks are eaten after being blanched, braised or steamed. (In Italy, the stems are often battered and fried.)

I have been told that the root is also edible after it is boiled. When I asked how it was typically served in Switzerland, I was told that it's paired with melted cheese. I steamed and used it as a substitute for Swiss chard.

In the U.S., cardoon is grown in northern California and can be found at Korean markets and specialty vegetable markets, such as Chelsea Market in Manhattan.

Ah, chocolate! Who doesn't dream of creamy, Swiss, milk chocolate? The Swiss are very proud of their reputation as world-class chocolatiers and use every occasion to celebrate it. It's customary to give chocolate as a gift when one is invited to dinner, or as a way to say "I love you" to your partner when visiting a chocolate shop on your way home from work.

While the global chocolate giant, Nestlé (makers of Nestlé's Crunch, Oh Henry!, Raisinets, etc.) originated in Switzerland, local artisan chocolate-makers own thriving businesses whose customers rely on them to make fine-quality, hand-made chocolate.

Frey (a subsidiary of Migros) makes my favorite chocolate, called "Noir Special," an extra-dark chocolate with a fondant filling. One chocolate ball weighs 12.5 grams

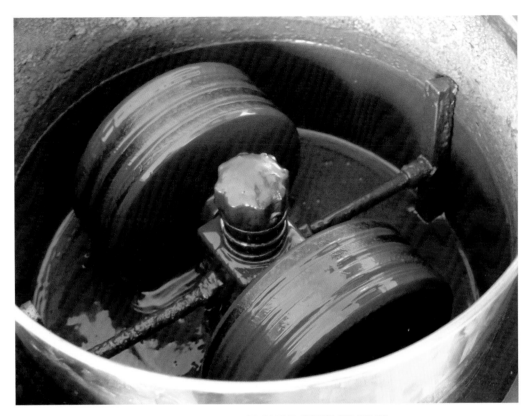

CONCHING MACHINE FOR MAKING CREAMY CHOCOLATE

(almost a half ounce) and contains 73 calories, five grams of sugar (about one teaspoon) and five-and-a-half grams of fat (about one teaspoon). If you eat only one a day, a small bag will last twenty days. Noir Special can be ordered online.

Fondant chocolate is the result of an invention of the "conching machine," a special mixer made just for chocolate by Rodolphe Lindt in 1879. Lindt added cocoa butter to chocolate liquor and created a new version of chocolate with a velvety smooth, fluid-like texture. In the same amount of Hershey's milk chocolate, you'll get an extra half-teaspoon of sugar.

THE SWISS STAPLES: YOGURT AND CHEESE

Switzerland is known for creamy yogurts and fresh cheeses made from the wholesome milk of contented Swiss dairy cows. Swiss-style yogurt is stirred so that the fruit is blended into the yogurt. Americans tend to favor yogurt with fruit on the bottom.

I've been told there's a Swiss law requiring a certain amount of bacterial culture be present in yogurt. The U.S. has a standard of identity for yogurt that offers a set of requirements in order for a product to be labeled "yogurt." Unfortunately, it does not specify any required amounts of culture be present in yogurt—just that it must contain a lactic acid-producing bacterium. Besides liking the taste, the main reason why we eat yogurt is to get the benefits of live cultures in our bellies. So wouldn't it make sense to make this a requirement?

Yogurt is high in protein, calcium and B vitamins. Those yogurts that contain live cultures, or probiotics, support the presence of good bacteria in your gut. Look for a *Live & Active Cultures* seal from the National Yogurt Association to insure that the yogurt has significant amounts of live and active cultures.

In Switzerland, mocha and coffee yogurts are popular flavors and my personal favorites. With the exception of Dannon's low-fat coffee and a "recently-launched" three-and-a-half ounce Chobani coffee with dark chocolate chips, it's hard to find this flavor of yogurt in the U.S. In Switzerland, it is difficult to find yogurts differentiated by fat content. Instead, you will see soy, lactose-free and organic varieties. In the U.S., I've noticed that low-fat yogurt is made with cultured nonfat milk and cream, rather than simply low-fat milk. U.S. companies often manipulate ingredients to optimize taste; all is apparently fair as long as the final fat content meets their health claims. When best quality ingredients are used, there is less need to manipulate and enhance flavor and texture.

Fresh cheeses are often called "un-aged" or "curd-style." Curdling milk with an enzyme or an acid and draining off the whey makes the cheeses. The curds that remain are molded into cheese. Common examples are ricotta, cottage and farmer cheeses.

Fresh cheeses are known for their ability to retain the flavor of fresh milk. That's why the fresh cheeses of Switzerland taste so good—they are created with whole-some Swiss milk! Fresh cheeses are high in water content, tend to be lower in fat and sodium, and must be handled like milk—always refrigerated. They are bland and work well combined with other foods in pastries, crêpes and spreads. For example, ricotta cheesecake is my favorite Italian pastry, especially when it's made with healthier, part-skim ricotta. See recipe in Part Three.

Fresh, natural, low-fat cheeses are staples of the Swiss diet. *Sérac*, of French origin, is a low-fat, ricotta-like cheese. Quark, of German origin, resembles a low-fat, soft, cream cheese with a consistency similar to Greek yogurt. It's a nice accompaniment to wild (or organic) smoked salmon that is not laden with unnaturally occurring nitrites and chemicals.

Magerquark (*mager* means "lean" in German) is a lower-fat version of quark and makes a perfect base for a creamy salad dressing or spread. Magerquark fruit cups are a healthy alternative to our pudding cups. You can make them by combining quark with fresh fruit in a blender. In the U.S., quark can be found in most natural food markets.

Fromage blanc, of French origin, means "white cheese," and is also known as *fromage frais* ("fresh cheese"). It's similar to quark—creamy and soft, made with cultured skim milk (sometimes cream is added), but originating in France.

All of these cheeses have fewer calories and less cholesterol than cream cheese and sour cream. Fromage blanc is served at the end of a meal, sometimes with added fruit, or is used in savory dishes to thicken sauces. I like to combine it with fresh herbs and use it as a spread on bread. It is also served with honey and called *fromage blanc au miel* or "white cheese with honey."

A TYPICAL DAY OF BLISSFUL EATING FOR THE SWISS

The typical start to a Swiss day is a minimal breakfast—a slice or two of hearty bread topped with a small amount of jam, marmalade, honey, cheese or butter, accompanied by coffee or tea. Kids tend to have cereal with hot or cold milk.

Lunches in Switzerland tend to be heavier than dinners. They are approached with a leisurely attitude and not rushed or wolfed down at a desk or between meetings. A lunch might consist of a small plate of pasta with a simple salad, or meat, potatoes and vegetables. The tradition of eating the largest meal at lunchtime comes from Swiss farm workers, who ate their largest meals early to give them fuel for their grueling days on the land.

Is it true that one should "eat breakfast like a king, lunch like a prince and dinner like a pauper?" It really depends on what works best for you. If you are hungriest at 4 p.m., it may be better for you to have four mini-meals each day—just enough to satisfy your hunger. There is conflicting data about whether or not eating more food early or late can affect weight control. However, if one doesn't eat enough during the day, there's a tendency to overeat at night to compensate. Then, food tends to sit in the stomach, potentially contributing to acid reflux and indigestion.

The Swiss often take a late afternoon break for a coffee or tea with a small pastry or half sandwich. Depending upon lunch, the evening meal might be a light supper, such as an omelet with a salad or antipasto in regions near Italy, or dried meats and a piece of fruit, cheese and bread.

It's not unusual to have a small piece of chocolate every day!

MYTHS AND TRUTHS ABOUT SWISS FOOD

• *Chocolate is part of the diet in Switzerland, because it's a heart-healthy food.*
  (MYTH)

Like yodeling, eating chocolate is part of the Swiss tradition. In terms of being heart-healthy, it is raw cocoa that is rich in flavonoids and benefits heart health, lowering blood pressure. Chocolate, which is made from cocoa beans, has added cocoa butter, sugar and, if it's milk chocolate, milk. Therefore, chocolate as you know it today is high in fat, sugar and calories.

In the case of chocolate, moderation is important. A small amount of high-quality dark chocolate can be satisfying and delicious, but don't believe the media hype calling it a "miracle food." Your healthiest choice is dark chocolate made with at least 70 percent cocoa.

• *The Swiss cheese you buy in America is made in Switzerland.*
  (MYTH)

What you know as "Swiss cheese," the one with the holes in it, is made in America, not Switzerland. Our Swiss version was invented to resemble Emmental, a cheese originally made in the Emme River Valley in west central Switzerland. Today Emmental cheese is also made in France, Germany and the U.S. When you buy cheese, always ask if it is domestic (made in the U.S.) or imported.

Switzerland makes over 450 types of cheese (but not cheddar or any orange-colored cheeses). The taste of cheese varies widely depending upon bacterial culture, the technique in its production, and the type and quality of milk. Even the same kind of cheese can taste different depending upon the diet of the cow, sheep or goat. A pasture-fed cow will produce milk with a unique taste based on the grasses, herbs and flowers of that pasture.

American cheese is typically made in highly automated factories. American cows are typically fed grains, hay and silage. Swiss law requires that cows go outside at least 20 days each month and seek their own food. Cheese from pastured cows taste very different than from cows fed silage.

By the way, the holes in Swiss cheeses are a result of the type of good bacteria used to turn the milk into cheese.

While Americans are trending more toward artisan cheeses produced by hand, using traditional craftsmanship from skilled cheesemakers, we still consume more processed cheese. This remains the number two source of dietary calcium. (Milk is number one.) Today, the U.S. has hundreds of artisan cheesemakers, a growing niche industry, to create flavors and styles that are uniquely American, such as Vermont Butter & Cheese Creamery's quark and fromage blanc.

• *The Swiss continue to rely on dairy as a staple of their diet.*
  (TRUTH)

Switzerland produces the world's best quality milk to sustain its thriving dairy industry. Compared to our dairies, the Swiss have smaller herd sizes, lower milk production and higher milk prices. Dairy producers adhere to strict quality-control guidelines to keep bacteria and antibiotics to a bare minimum; otherwise, they must pay steep fines. The dairy industry's goal is to keep their cows and their products healthy.

As a result, milk, cheese and yogurt are a big part of Switzerland's high-quality food system. Nutritionally, dairy foods are good sources of protein, zinc, B vitamins, and calcium, which help build and maintain strong bones. The stronger your bones, the less likely it is that you'll suffer from osteoporosis later in life.

The conventional dairy industry in our country is improving, but for now I would choose organically produced, hormone-free dairy products. For those wanting to lose weight, low-fat dairy products will help them get and stay slim. These products actually contain more calcium than their full-fat counterparts. Why? Because when the fat is removed, what remains is the calcium-rich part.

Research supports that low-fat dairy products, with their balance of calcium, magnesium, protein and other nutrients, as part of a healthy diet, can prevent heart disease, diabetes and stroke. Aim for three servings per day, such as one cup of fat-free milk or six ounces of low-fat yogurt. If you are lactose intolerant, choose lactose-free milk and/or four ounces of yogurt, which are generally well tolerated. Some individuals with lactose intolerance can eat cheese, while others cannot. Lactose is primarily in the whey, not the curds. A cheesemaker drains the whey from the curds (with the exception of some soft cheese like ricotta). Aged cheeses are low in moisture and low in lactose. Some people tolerate goat's milk over cow's milk, but that usually has to do with the fact that goat-milk fat is easier to digest.

About one in five people in Switzerland, and one out of three in the U.S. are affected by lactose intolerance—one's inability to tolerate the milk sugar, or lactose. Sufferers

41

cannot produce enough of the enzyme lactase which breaks down lactose, and the symptoms can be very uncomfortable: bloating, gas, diarrhea and pain in the lower belly.

PUTTING THE SECRETS OF THE SWISS DIET TO WORK FOR YOU

✓ *Drink water, herbal tea and mineral water throughout the day. Eight cups is a good goal. It helps keep your tummy full and your body well hydrated.*

✓ *Consume three servings daily (six to eight ounces per serving) of low-fat milk, yogurt and kefir for weight loss, to prevent osteoporosis and to control blood pressure. Opt for organic, hormone-free brands. If you cannot tolerate milk, choose almond, rice, soy or other dairy alternatives enriched with calcium and fortified with vitamin D.*

✓ *Eat one to two servings of dairy for protein each day. One serving equals three egg whites, or one ounce of reduced fat cheese, or ¼ cup fresh cheese, such as part-skim ricotta, farmer cheese, cottage cheese and quark.*

✓ *Indulge in as much pure (organic) cocoa as your heart desires, or have a small square of dark chocolate—at least 70 percent cocoa—once a day.*

✓ *Choose fermented and cultured foods, which can aid digestion.*

✓ *Stay active daily, even if it means just taking a 15-minute walk twice a day.*

✓ *Practice being a "locavore" (someone who chooses locally produced food).*

✓ *Instead of thinking about what you can't eat, think about all the natural-food options that are available.*

✓ *Take pleasure in planning your dinner. Prepare your meals with an eye-appealing presentation and eat mostly at home. Be sure to use a plate, sit at the table, and enjoy the company of family and friends.*

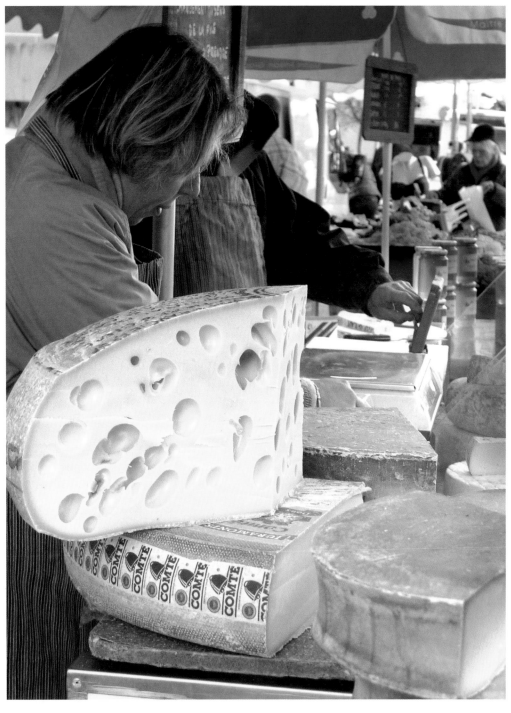

EMMENTAL (OR EMMENTALER) CHEESE ORIGINATED FROM EMMENTAL, SWITZERLAND, AT A FARMERS MARKET IN GENEVA

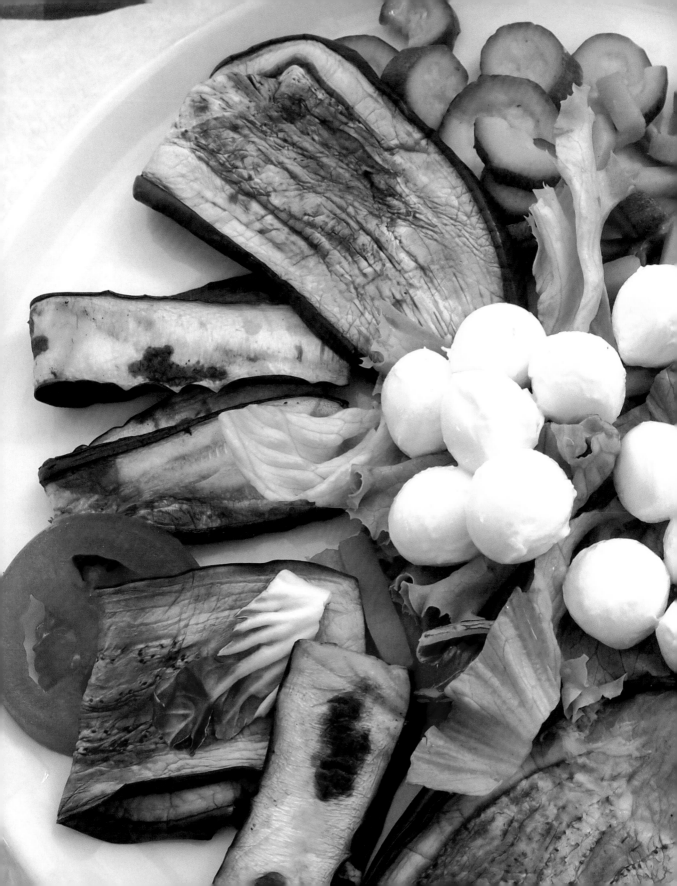

Chapter 3

THE SECRETS
OF THE
ITALIAN DIET

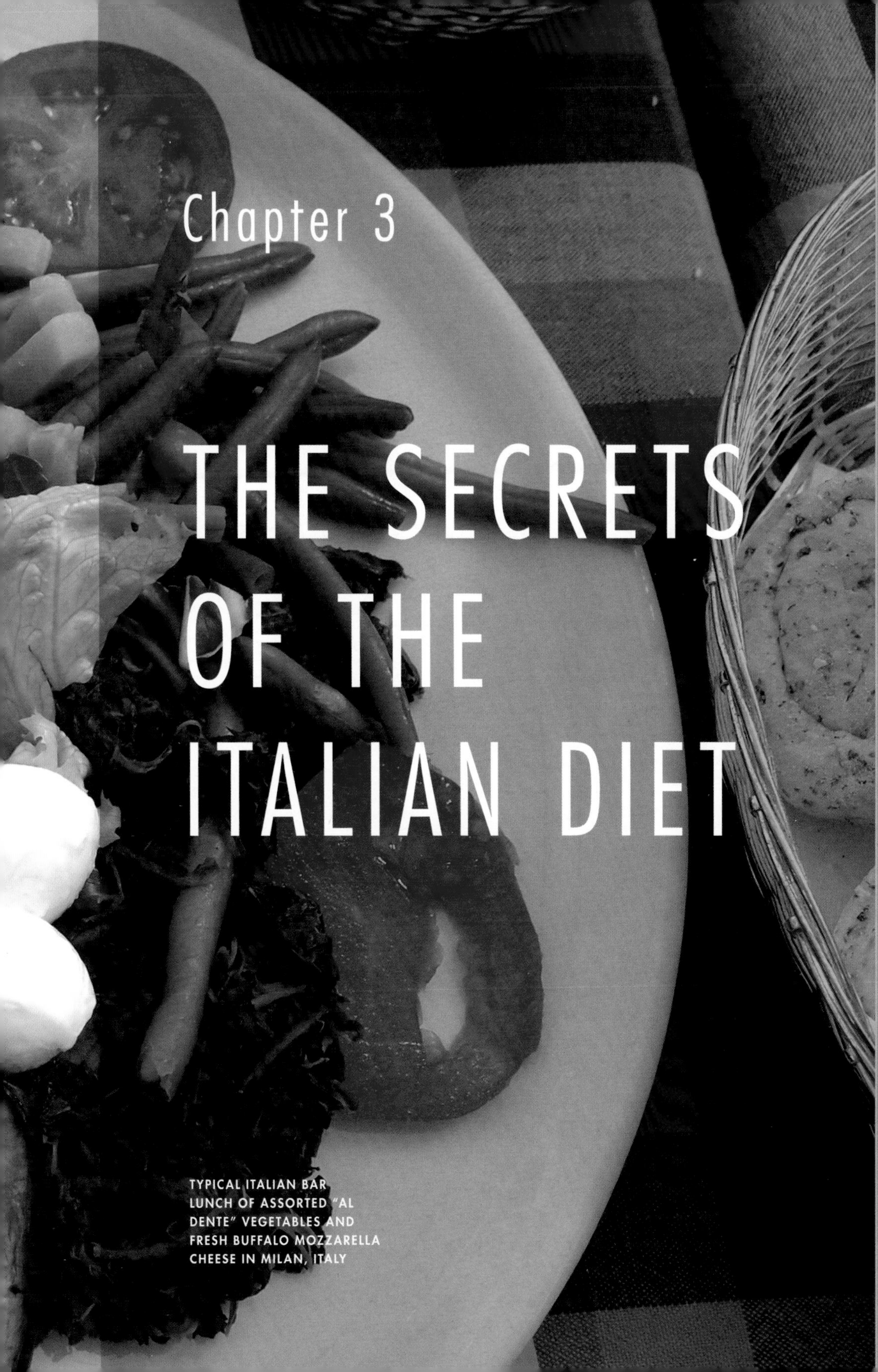

TYPICAL ITALIAN BAR
LUNCH OF ASSORTED "AL
DENTE" VEGETABLES AND
FRESH BUFFALO MOZZARELLA
CHEESE IN MILAN, ITALY

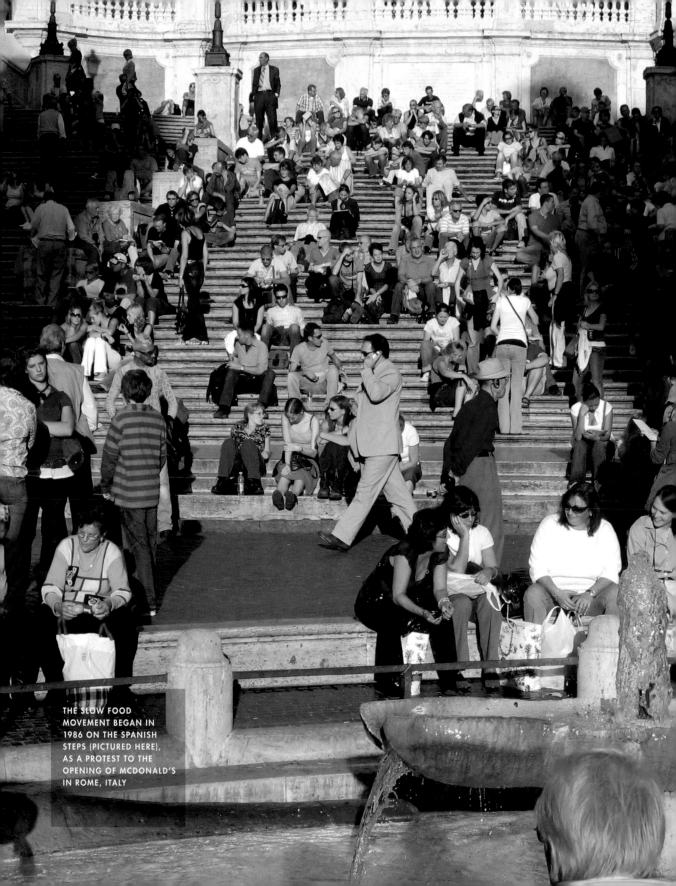

THE SLOW FOOD
MOVEMENT BEGAN IN
1986 ON THE SPANISH
STEPS (PICTURED HERE),
AS A PROTEST TO THE
OPENING OF MCDONALD'S
IN ROME, ITALY

talians are as passionate about food as they are about each other! If you go into a restaurant in Italy, you'll be struck with how much Italians enjoy their meals. Everyone is engaged in conversation, laughing and telling stories, and the meals can go on for hours. It's a time for sharing, bonding and enjoying food and each other.

In contrast, mealtime in faster-paced countries such as the U.S. can be a solitary business, where an addiction to smart phones or TV programs trumps the desire to connect with others—even at dinner.

It's no surprise that Italian food is America's favorite cuisine—but did you know it *could* slim your waistline and boost your health? Italy ranks number two among European countries boasting the longest life spans. Of course, you have to eat like a "real Italian," which does not include the typical American thick-crusted doughy pizza oozing with salty and highly processed mozzarella cheese.

Instead, find a pizzeria that specializes in authentic Neapolitan pizza. It should be made with a thin crust and the freshest ingredients, including basil, tomato and buffalo mozzarella cheese, and baked in a wood-burning oven.

ITALY: ORGANIC, YES—FAST FOOD, NOT SO FAST!

Surrounded by the Mediterranean Sea, this peninsular country has access to a wide variety of fish, and every town, village or city has abundant fresh pasta and vegetables. There are differences, depending on whether you live in the north or the south, but the principles of the Italian diet remain the same: fresh, local, organic ingredients are plentiful, and carbohydrates like pasta, polenta, risotto and bread are a staple at the table.

Italy has the largest certified organic food industry in Europe. It is also an important and growing sector for exports, mainly to Germany, Japan and the U.S. In fact, both Canada and the U.S. import more than half of Italy's organic (biologic) wine. The most common organic products are grains, olives, fruit, vegetables, citrus, vineyards and livestock. (Poultry production has recently seen steep growth.)

Italy's standards are so high; they do not accept U.S. products unless they are certified by the European Union, which controls organic labeling. Italian schools have commendably adopted organic meals for their school cafeterias. In 2010, there were 872 organic Italian school cafeterias—superb!

The Italians recognized that the influence of fast food was not good for their people, and Italy became the first country to start what is known as the "Slow Food movement." It all started when McDonald's opened its first restaurant in 1986 in Rome. Although fast food was unpopular at that time in Italy, McDonald's proved to be so popular that it created a mob scene on opening day. Young people were quickly hooked, and adults recognized the inherent danger of this fast food phenomenon.

That same year, an Italian named Carlo Petrini began the "Slow Food movement." His goal: to preserve traditional ways of eating and produce locally grown foods that benefited the eco-system. (See Appendix for more about Carlo Petrini and the Slow Food movement.) Since then, the movement has taken off and is now active in 150 countries around the world, including here in the United States. Now, thanks to followers of this movement, there is increasing support for local food artisans, a revival of traditional food production, and more farmers markets springing up in big cities, as well as small towns.

And in Italy, while some might go for the occasional McDonald's burger, it's just a cheap, quick diversion from their old favorite, the *panini* sandwich.

In Italy, panino *is the word for a sandwich made from bread other than sliced bread. Panini now refers to a pressed sandwich.*

LAYNE'S ITALIAN FAVORITES

My favorite Italian cuisine comes from the south of Italy, which features fresh and cooked tomato sauces, fresh ricotta and mozzarella cheeses, peppers, olives, artichokes, oranges, figs, eggplants, zucchini, capers and fish like anchovies, sardines and tuna. My Sicilian girlfriend, Nadia, raves about the fresh ricotta from her hometown of Ragusa, sold at 1.5 euros (about $1.95) per pound. Nadia, born and raised in Ragusa, dislikes garlic and swears that Italians do not *always* cook with garlic, and when they do it's sparingly. For example, Nadia says, "Many of the red sauces have onion, but not garlic. And not every pasta dish should be smothered with grated pecorino or Parmigiano cheese, especially dishes prepared with fish, mushrooms, olives and capers."

One of my best memories is traveling with my oldest son, Ben, and eating pizza in Pompeii, near Naples. Neapolitan pizza comes from the city of Naples, where pizza originated. A pizza here is about 10-inches across, perfect for one or two persons, and should be eaten right away. This pizza has the right balance of crust, sauce and cheese, without emphasizing one single component. A true Neapolitan 10-inch pizza holds about two-and-a-half ounces of cheese, two-and-a-half ounces of sauce and five ounces of dough. This equals 880 calories.

In contrast, the same pizza in the U.S. holds about four ounces of cheese (double), two-and-a-half ounces of sauce and eight ounces of dough. This equals 1,400 calories.

What a difference! American pizza is known to sit out all day and still seem fresh because of all the dough stabilizers added to the flour.

Another famous Italian dish I love is referred to as "scaloppini," thinly sliced (or pounded) chicken or veal, lightly dipped in flour, sautéed in a small amount of olive oil and finished with red or white wine. In Italy, a typical slice of homemade veal scaloppini weighs two ounces, contains 230 calories and nine grams of fat. The American version is heavily breaded, deep-fried and two or three times as large, amounting to over 500 calories and 24 grams of fat.

In Italy, pasta is a staple in almost every household. It's traditionally served as a small starter course the size of a small salad bowl. It would be no larger than one cup cooked, about 200 calories and one to two grams of fat. In addition to the pasta, a small portion of tomato sauce gently coats the pasta, adding another 25 calories.

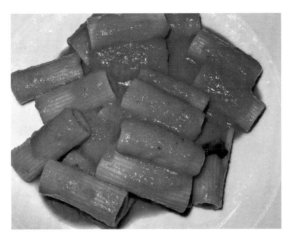

ONE CUP OF COOKED ITALIAN RIGATONI PASTA WITH TOMATO SAUCE

Compare this to our present American version of pasta, which averages two cups cooked, drowning in sauce and amounting to over 500 calories and five grams of fat. Unfortunately, instead of chopping up fresh tomatoes for sauce, we tend to use pre-made tomato sauce, which usually includes a heavy dose of salt. Tomato sauces in jars average about 500 milligrams of sodium per half cup.

THE GLUTEN-FREE QUESTION

Today, there is a lot of discussion about celiac disease and gluten intolerance. Yet no one really knows what's causing it, and whether it is just a fad or if we are indeed developing a greater intolerance to gluten. "Gluten" refers to the proteins found in all grains, but people with celiac disease react unfavorably to the glutens found in wheat, barley, rye and oats that are contaminated by wheat.

Italian pasta is made with durum wheat, which is grown both in Europe and the U.S., and is a natural hybrid (a cross between two wild species that occurred in the wild, as opposed to being man-made). Since this is a type of wheat, it is off limits to those with celiac disease.

One explanation for gluten intolerance is that over the years, wild grasses naturally crossed with ancient wheat strains. Modern man then hybridized them, and the result may have been a greater degree of digestive intolerance.

There's another theory that suggests we are responding to the results of "refining" wheat, which makes it devoid of nutrients, low in fiber and an overall poor fit for our digestive tracts.

In my opinion, the crux of the problem is the unhealthy American diet laden with processed foods, sugar and hydrogenated fats mixed with factory-farmed meats containing antibiotics. This combination definitely results in poor gut health, since this diet lacks the good bacteria that keep our digestive systems working properly.

Italian pasta is admittedly high in gluten, because it's made from hard durum wheat, which is also used to make semolina flour. So what to do? Eat wholesome, organic and less-processed foods like our European friends do to get your figure, and your digestion, back to normal. Then, choose more natural grains (sprouted, ancient and whole). For now, if you don't have celiac disease or gluten intolerance, enjoy authentic Italian pasta on the right-sized plate!

ITALIAN DIETARY GUIDELINES

Here are the Italian dietary guidelines based on the recommendations from the Italian Ministry of Health:

1. Watch your weight and be active. Walk often and take part in sports and other lifestyle activities such as walking, hiking and swimming.

2. Eat more complex carbohydrates: cereals, vegetables, tubers and fruit. Health-conscious Italians eat whole grains and enjoy whole-wheat pasta. Yet they aren't quite ready to give up pasta made from white flour!

3. Use high-quality fats in limited amounts. These include cold-pressed extra-virgin olive oil, high in monounsaturated fat. However, too much of any fat can cause weight problems, because fats carry nine calories per gram, compared to carbohydrates or proteins, which are four calories per gram.

4. Enjoy your sugars and sweets, but in moderation. Italians love their biscotti, gelato and fresh-squeezed orange juice. The right portions are four ounces of juice in the morning, one scoop of gelato or one or two biscotti for dessert.

5. Drink plenty of water, at least eight eight-ounce glasses of water a day. Italians love mineral water, both flat and sparkling. They know it's important to drink water with meals and throughout the day.

6. Salt? The less, the better. When cooking pasta, Italians add salt to the water, but they don't add additional salt to the cooked pasta or to the sauce! (Pasta absorbs salt from the cooking water.)

    Our bodies need only 180 to 500 milligrams of salt per day. According to the Institute of Medicine, the limit for Americans is 2,300 milligrams per day. Half our population has health restrictions and should not exceed 1,500 milligrams per day. Since the 1970s, the amount of sodium in our food has increased, and because we are eating more food than ever, we are consuming more sodium.

    The majority of the sodium we consume is from processed and restaurant foods. Only a small portion is used in cooking or added at the table. One teaspoon of salt has 2,300 milligrams of sodium!

7. Alcoholic drinks are fine, but in limited amounts. Italians sip their wine slowly, and limit their intake to one or two four-ounce glasses a day. Prosecco, a delicious Italian sparkling wine, has fewer calories than regular wine—five calories less per ounce—so it's a good way to save calories while still enjoying yourself! (Even though in most of Italy the legal drinking age is 16, everybody is forbidden from being in a state of inebriation.)

8. Don't limit yourself to pasta and meats. Instead, vary your food choices to benefit from a variety of nutrients. For example, instead of wheat pasta, try cornmeal polenta or whole-grain rice. Today, there are wheat-free pastas made from quinoa, rice, potato and other grains. Vary your choices for vegetables and fruits, choosing seasonal and local varieties when available.

9. If you have special dietary needs, check with your nutritionist or physician. Seek nutritional advice if you are pregnant, lactating or have other special dietary needs. Those with chronic illnesses, such as diabetes, high cholesterol, hypertension and certain cancers, may need further dietary modification in order to control these diseases.

10. Remember, ensuring that your food is safe is *your* responsibility. Follow food safety guidelines, such as washing your hands before and after handling food,

refrigerating food promptly, cooking at the right temperature, and avoiding cross-contaminating foods.

Don't leave perishable food out at room temperature for more than two hours.

THE ITALIAN FOOD PYRAMID

The traditional Italian Food Pyramid is divided into six food groups to be eaten daily. Beginning from the base, the divisions are:

1. Fruits and vegetables (five to six portions)
2. Bread, pasta, rice, biscuits, potato (four to five portions)
3. Oil and fats (two to three portions)

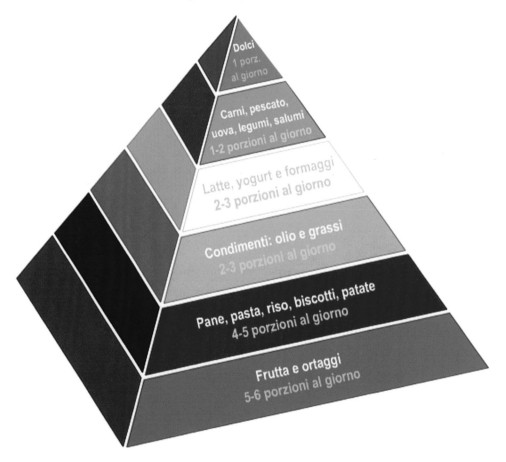

Dolci
1 porz.
al giorno

Carni, pescato,
uova, legumi, salumi
1-2 porzioni al giorno

Latte, yogurt e formaggi
2-3 porzioni al giorno

Condimenti: olio e grassi
2-3 porzioni al giorno

Pane, pasta, riso, biscotti, patate
4-5 porzioni al giorno

Frutta e ortaggi
5-6 porzioni al giorno

Source: www.piramidealimentare.it

4. Milk, yogurt and cheese (two to three portions)
5. Meat, fish, eggs, legumes and processed meats (one to two portions)
6. Sweets (one portion)

Interestingly, our newest USDA food guide (2011), "MyPlate," falls short on advice about proper portion sizes, and U.S. food labels fail to offer uniform serving sizes. In the European Union (EU), food labels are required to provide nutrition information based on 100 grams of the product, no matter what it is. With lack of guidance, portion-size confusion and the food industry supersizing our food, we need to regain control. We can learn from the Italians how to enjoy authentic, properly portioned food and carbohydrate-count instinctually.

WHAT *ABOUT* THE TRADITIONAL MEDITERRANEAN DIET?

You cannot talk about Italian dietary guidelines without bringing up the Mediterranean diet. First publicized in 1945, the concept of the Mediterranean diet (named for the Mediterranean Sea) was originally regarded as the reason why *southern* Italians lived longer and had lower rates of heart disease than other countries.

The diet focused on consumption of large amounts of olive oil, legumes, whole grains, fruits, vegetables, moderate-to-high amounts of fish, moderate amounts of dairy (mostly as cheese and yogurt) and poultry and moderate amounts of wine. Meat was to be relegated to the "occasional" category.

Back then, in 1945, the Mediterranean diet was a diet of poverty—it wasn't a choice. As soon as people had more money, meat consumption increased. Today, three generations later, Italian children are enamored with American fast food, and the Mediterranean diet is out of favor. Fresh fruit, vegetables, seafood and good-quality olive oil are more expensive than processed foods, even in Italy!

Health professionals and organizations, like the Slow Food movement in Italy, are doing all they can to reverse this trend towards fast food. In Italy, as in other countries, childhood obesity is rising. There is a push for the younger generation to rediscover culinary traditions and get back to eating locally produced food.

------

*A person is considered obese when his/her BMI (body mass index)
is greater than or equal to 30. BMI is a measure of body fat
calculated from one's height and current weight.*

Italians do not want to lose their ranking of second on the list of European countries that boast the longest life spans! Later, in Chapter 5, I will expand on why going *Beyond the Mediterranean Diet* works.

Now, let's see how Italy's native cuisine and love for life translate into a healthy diet and longer life spans!

THE HEALTHY ITALIAN DIET

Italy is much more than its pasta, pizza and mozzarella. It's known for family cooking, with recipes passed down from revered grandmothers rather than from celebrity chefs. Kids race home from school to enjoy freshly made lunches (or savor organic lunches available at school). It's rare to hear anyone obsess about dieting. Food is an essential part of family life one shares with loved ones.

As part of the generous, outgoing nature of Italians, in restaurants waiters will leave full bottles of wine or after-dinner *digestivos* (liquors, usually enhanced with herbs to promote digestion) on the table, with no fear that customers will overindulge. This is an example of the unspoken relationship of trust and responsibility among Italians.

A key difference between the Italian diet and the American diet may be summed up in one word—sugar. Italians don't eat much sugar. On average, only eight percent of their total calories come from sugar, compared with 18 percent in the U.S. As an example, Italians drink 57 cups of fruit juice (a naturally sugary drink) per person every year compared to 181 cups in the U.S.!

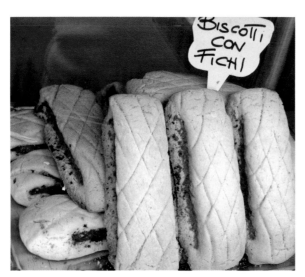

FANCY ITALIAN BISCOTTI MADE WITH FIG

This increased amount of sugar in the U.S., especially from high fructose corn syrup (HFCS), certainly helps explain why obesity and possibly Type 2 diabetes are soaring. A 2012 study by University of Oxford and University of Southern California researchers reveals that countries using high fructose corn syrup in their food supply had a 20 percent higher prevalence of diabetes than countries that did not use it. HFCS is sweeter than ordinary sugar and provides processed foods with a more consistent brown color.

Italians favor fruit, which may be marinated in wine or balsamic vinegar, for dessert. This is certainly healthier than the American apple, berry, or peach "crumble," which is then topped with lots of butter and sugar, or that store-bought pie sweetened with corn syrup.

Biscotto, a twice-baked almond biscuit, is another popular Italian dessert; it is common to dip a biscotto into the last bit of wine, as the cookie itself is dry. A biscotto makes a great complement to a drink, whether it's wine, tea or coffee.

One Italian biscotto averages 70 calories and three grams of fat.

Italians often skip dessert at the dinner table in favor of an evening stroll to pick up a small cup of gelato, served with the universal teeny spoon so the treat lasts longer. Gelato has less fat than ice cream, which is between 10 percent and 19 percent butterfat, while gelato contains only three to 10 percent butterfat. (Sorbet has zero butterfat, since it's made of frozen fruit juice, sugar and water.)

Italians are proud of many world-class "authentic" food products named after where they are produced. Two familiar examples include:

Parmigiano-Reggiano (Parmesan) cheese, made from cow's milk. It has a nutty flavor and is so potent, just a small amount can go a long way! One tablespoon of grated Parmesan has 22 calories, two grams of protein, 70 milligrams of calcium and just one gram of fat, and it's a low-lactose food for those who are lactose-intolerant. Its salty taste also makes it a good substitute for salt. So besides sprinkling freshly grated Parmesan on pasta, try it on a baked potato, salad greens and soups. Real Parmigiano-Reggiano *must be* imported from a designated region of Italy and legally cannot be made anywhere else. *Grana Padano,* a "close cousin" in taste and texture, is also made in Italy.

Traditional *Modena* balsamic vinegar and its less-expensive "modern" balsamic vinegar from Modena, Italy, are different from U.S.-made balsamic vinegar. The traditional version is made by pressing two varieties of grapes and is aged for a minimum of 12 years in seven different wood barrels. The modern balsamic vinegar of Modena is produced with a similar technique but only aged up to three years. If it's aged more than three years, it wins the label "aged."

Domestic balsamic vinegar (produced in the U.S.) is made from wine vinegar blended with grape juice or grape *must*, which contains the skin, seeds and stems of grapes. Caramel is sometimes added for color stability. Although caramel coloring *sounds* innocent, there are varieties known to contain ammonium and sulfites. Not all that appealing, is it!

Balsamic vinegars range from 14 to 20 calories per tablespoon. Almost all balsamic and red wine vinegars contain a minute amount of lead, most likely absorbed by the grapes from naturally occurring lead in the soil. One would have to consume one to two cups of balsamic vinegar per day in order to be affected by the lead, so it's nothing much to worry about it.

Italians report that one or two tablespoons of balsamic vinegar provide relief from heartburn.

FOOD SHOPPING, ITALIAN STYLE

Corner food shops, fruit and vegetable vendors, and neighborhood butchers may create an idyllic Italian tableau, but in reality, most families go shopping once a week at the local supermarket or *supermercato.* An important health rule when food shopping in Italy is "You Cannot Touch Unpackaged Foods," such as fresh fruits and vegetables. Instead, supermarkets provide disposable gloves for customers, placed near the produce counters.

In all three countries (Switzerland, Italy and France) there are two important food-shopping practices:

1. Shoppers are responsible for weighing and printing out price labels for fruits and vegetables, then heading to the checkout line to pay.
2. Shoppers bring their own bags or are expected to pay for each one. Progressive Italy actually outlawed plastic bags in 2011.

Both practices impart greater responsibility to the consumer when handling food, which helps create a respectful relationship between shoppers and their food purveyors.

Most of the supermarkets in Italy have butchers, fishmongers and a cheese and charcuterie counter. Often they have a bakery and a prepared foods or *gastronomia* section for local specialties. While there are lots of shelves featuring bottled mineral waters and a variety of dried pastas, there are far fewer featuring breakfast cereals and packaged foods, because there is less demand for them.

Most milk is sold in sterile boxes, rather than bottles. It is processed under ultra-high temperatures, does not require refrigeration prior to opening, and has an unopened

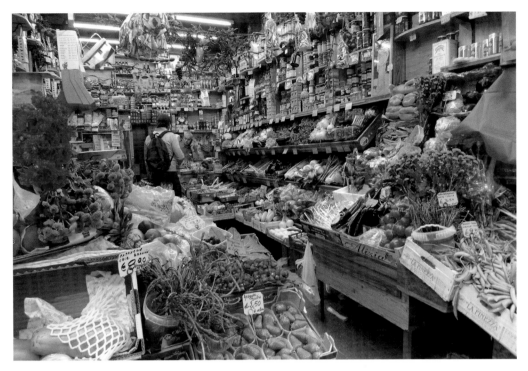

FRUIT AND VEGETABLE SHOP IN THE BRERA DISTRICT OF MILAN, ITALY

shelf life of six to nine months. Eggs are also found on shelves near the coolers, which are packed with fresh pasta and regional cheeses.

The wine and spirits aisle offers a wide choice of products, including *limoncello*, an Italian liqueur made from the lemons of southern Italy and served chilled as an after-dinner *digestivo.* There are producers now in the U.S. making *limoncello* from California-grown lemons. While it is often too sweet, there are a number of excellent handcrafted and organic brands. Just be sure you avoid any that have added artificial coloring or flavoring.

If you're in Italy, you'll find shops that sell fresh fruits and vegetables exclusively. These are called *frutta e verdure.* The shopkeeper will give you a plastic bag to fill or will fill it for you. (Remember, no touching the produce!)

If you want to indicate how many pieces you would like to buy, start with holding up your thumb as number one. For two, hold up your thumb and pointer finger, and so on.

The fruits and vegetables in Italy are some of the best I've ever eaten, and the south grows some of the tastiest oranges, tomatoes and lemons in the world. If you're lucky, you'll get to taste a real *San Marzano* plum tomato. They are the only tomatoes allowed on pizza made in Naples, the world's best and original pizza! They are also the most coveted canned tomatoes found on U.S. grocery shelves.

SPECIALTY FOODS, ITALIAN-STYLE

The beauty of Italian cooking is that you only need a few ingredients to create flavorful, satisfying dishes. Besides pasta, pizza and scaloppini, let's explore a few other specialty foods that make Italian cuisine beloved the world over.

Pesto sauce comes from northern Italy and tastes delicious on almost everything. It is usually made from basil leaves, but can also be made with spinach, cilantro or parsley—any type of fragrant, herbaceous greens. These are ground to a paste with olive oil, garlic, pine nuts and Parmesan cheese. Bright green and bursting with garlicky flavor, this is a treat on top of fresh pasta, chicken, vegetables or even as a spread on toast with chopped Roma tomatoes. To lower the fat content, leave out the nuts and replace some of the oil with lemon juice or water.

Focaccia, popular throughout Italy, is yeast bread baked in flat sheet pans, essentially made from the same ingredients as pizza dough. It's chewy and moist, usually drizzled with olive oil and can have a variety of toppings on it or be served plain. I like it covered with chunks of vine-ripened tomatoes and sprinkled with chopped, fresh rosemary.

Pasta Fagioli, a soup of pasta and beans, usually meatless, started out as a humble, inexpensive peasant dish but is now served everywhere. The pasta shape is similar to elbow macaroni, and the beans are either cooked cannellini or *borlotti*, also known as "cranberry beans."

To make this soup, begin by sautéing onions and garlic in a small amount of olive oil, then add spices, tomato sauce (and/or vegetable broth), and finally add the beans and pasta. I like adding freshly chopped kale. Either way, this soup makes a complete high-fiber, high-protein, vegetarian meal. The best part is sopping up the last traces of the soup with a piece of hearty Italian sourdough bread.

Chicken Cacciatore ("hunter's chicken") has many varieties, based on the region. Basically, it is prepared with tomatoes, onions, herbs, bell peppers and a cut-up chicken. Sometimes white or red wine is added, along with a bay leaf and carrots, and then cooked on a slow simmer to develop the rich flavors. To make a leaner version, remove the skin of the chicken before cooking.

Spaghetti Puttanesca ("whore's-style spaghetti") is a popular pasta dish from southern Italy, circa 1950s. It's made with olives, capers, garlic and tomatoes. It can be salty, so to reduce the salt, rinse the olives and capers and use freshly chopped tomatoes or buy "no salt added" canned tomatoes. To increase fiber, choose whole-wheat or whole-grain spaghetti. "Whole" is better than "white," because it's less processed and is a natural source of fiber, selenium, potassium, magnesium and B vitamins.

Insalata Caprese (salad in the style of Capri, an island of Italy) is a salad of sliced tomatoes, fresh buffalo mozzarella (made from the milk of water buffalo) and basil leaves, often dressed with olive oil. This is usually an antipasto (meaning "before the food") served before the main dish. To make it slenderizing, use part-skim mozzarella and forgo the olive oil, using balsamic vinegar instead. If you are watching salt intake, go for a no-salt-added mozzarella.

In Italy, fresh mozzarella is eaten immediately after it's made. So to refresh store-bought mozzarella, take it out of the refrigerator and soak it for about an hour in a warm, lightly salted milk bath, then serve.

Involtini means "a small bite of food" that is raw or cooked, consisting of an outer layer that wraps around a filling. Examples are a wrapper of prosciutto around a piece of cantaloupe or a thin slice of grilled eggplant around a dollop of fresh ricotta, simmering in marinara sauce. Mmmm! Getting hungry?

Kaki fruit, which has a short, late-autumn season, is the Italian sweet variety of a persimmon, high in vitamins A and C. There are many varieties of persimmons grown around the world. The Italian variety has fragile skin and a pudding-like texture. It is not the astringent type commonly found in the U.S. The Italian kaki is sweet and juicy, with a hint of cantaloupe flavor.

Europeans consume a lot of this fruit, because it's too fragile to export long distances. For a similar taste experience, ask your supermarket for non-astringent types (also called "non-puckers") grown in California.

Roasted sweet chestnuts throughout Europe are fresh, perfectly roasted and easy to pop out of their scored shells and into your mouth. They are grown in a protected geographic area of northern Tuscany, specifically designated for

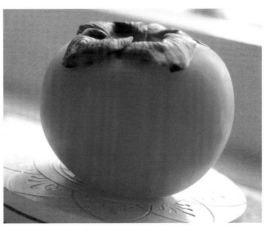

KAKI FRUIT FROM ITALY

59

chestnut production. Unlike the floury, moldy taste we often experience here in the U.S., these chestnuts are sweet, with subtle notes of hazelnut and the aroma of fresh bread.

Chestnuts are naturally gluten-free, low in calories, high in fiber, folic acid and vitamin C, and contain trace minerals and a small amount of monounsaturated fat.

I love the aroma of chestnuts being freshly roasted in covered huts along European city streets. For a similar experience, try domestic chestnuts from Washington State. (You can buy them online and have them shipped.) You can also find organic, cooked and shelled chestnuts packaged in natural food stores.

Chestnuts are one of the most popular street food snacks in Europe, roasted in sheds right in front of your eyes. Ten roasted chestnuts contain 206 calories, 1.85 grams of fat, 4.3 grams of fiber, two milligrams of sodium and are an excellent source of vitamin C.

Fresh, earthy *white truffles* (edible underground mushrooms) are celebrated during the short autumn season in northern Italy. White truffles are too delicate to be cooked and are so delicious shaved over pasta, you won't need Parmesan cheese!

For a similar experience, try white truffle-infused olive oil. It's also a good (and less expensive) way to extend the truffle season. The advantage of using flavored oils is that less goes a long way, resulting in a burst of flavor with fewer calories.

Coffee in Italy is divine, and the only time I drink coffee is when I'm in Italy. Italian baristas make the perfect skinny cappuccino, called *cappuccino con latte scremato.* This is probably the only country in Europe where you won't easily find a Starbucks. Yet CEO Howard Schultz, who enjoyed the baristas in the cafés throughout Italy, conceived the idea of Starbucks while visiting there in 1983. When Starbucks wanted to come to Italy, Italians recognized that this endangered the thousands of local coffee shops around the country.

While there may be one in Florence (for the tourists), there is no national presence for Starbucks. The Italians are proud of their own excellent foods, including coffee, and are unwilling to cede control to foreign interlopers.

A TYPICAL DAY OF BLISSFUL EATING FOR THE ITALIANS

For breakfast, or *colazione,* many Italians start with *brioche* and coffee or cappuccino. A brioche is the Italian version of a *croissant,* except that it's puffy and resembles a popover. A French croissant is crispy and flaky and has more butter than a brioche, which

60

has a softer texture and a golden hue. Breakfast cereal is uncommon in Italy, except for children, who enjoy it with hot chocolate, or cold or hot milk.

Italians love to make fresh orange juice every day by pressing two fresh oranges using an old-fashioned juice press. It's a great way to get natural vitamin C and burn calories! In Italy, it's rare for anyone to drink orange juice from a carton.

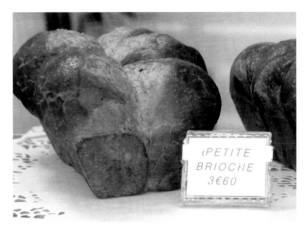

ITALIAN BRIOCHE AT A FRENCH PÂTISSERIE

Americans think they are being healthy by consuming gallons of orange juice, but do you know what's lurking in "100 percent pure" and "not from concentrate" Florida orange juice? The juice actually contains industry-produced flavor packs used during processing to ensure that every carton of juice tastes the same!

In mid-morning, a hungry Italian might have a cappuccino with a bread roll or panino.

Lunch, or *pranzo,* is considered the most important and the largest meal of the day. A traditional lunch consists of a first course, such as a vegetable-based soup or a small portion of thinly sliced cured meat. The second course is often a half-portion of pasta, and a third course features a small portion of meat, poultry or fish with vegetables. Salad is served with, or at the end of, the meal to aid in digestion.

In Italy, unless named otherwise like Insalata Caprese *salad is simply salad greens—arugula (also known as rocket) is most popular—sometimes served with other raw vegetables like tomatoes, onions and carrots, and dressed with olive oil, vinegar (or lemon) and herbs.*

In France, mâche (also known as lamb's lettuce) is a popular salad green.

During the meal, mineral water and wine are offered. The meal ends with espresso and/or a digestive alcoholic drink and biscotti. Today, because of a faster-paced lifestyle, Italians often opt for two courses rather than three.

61

Until recently, most Italians enjoyed lunch at home with family. This was often a one-course meal—pasta with a green salad and fruit, or a green salad with baked fish and potatoes. Despite the worldwide trend toward being busy 24/7, Italians still have a traditional two-to-three-hour, multi-course, family lunch on Sundays.

A snack, or *merenda*, is eaten around 4 p.m. This might consist of a piece of bread, fruit, or yogurt, and is usually waiting for the kids when they arrive home from school.

A prelude to dinner, or *aperitivo*, is served between 6:30 p.m. and 7:30 p.m. It's a tradition of snacking and socializing to wind down after a hard day's work. It started in northern Italy and has recently spread to the rest of the peninsula. A "bar" will host this event as a pre-dinner social with a free buffet of both hot and cold dishes, accompanying a single drink order, even if it's not alcoholic. Whether you order a cocktail drink or mineral water, rest assured that you will be overcharged to make up for the "all-you-can-eat" bar buffet. Still, the *aperitivo* is a hip, trendy way to begin a special evening.

When Italians want to cut calories without sacrificing pleasure, they may choose to drink *Prosecco*, a sparkling white wine (Italy's version of champagne) with less alcohol than traditional wine. It contains 20 calories per ounce, compared to 25 calories per ounce for an average red or white wine. Americans may dismiss this small difference in calories, yet such small changes have been proven to affect long-term weight loss success.

Certainly, a four-ounce glass of Prosecco at 80 calories is very appealing, compared to the American five-ounce "big pour" of wine tipping the scale at 125 calories.

A popular Italian cocktail is a Bellini, a mix of two ounces of Prosecco and two ounces of fresh peach puree. Prosecco is available here in the U.S. In fact, it's the third most important export market (after Germany and Switzerland) for the 160 million or so bottles produced in Italy every year. And it's less expensive than champagne!

Dinner, or *cena*, is usually a light meal of soup or salad, risotto, pasta or leftovers. Italians do their "carbohydrate counting" intuitively: if they eat meat, poultry or fish for lunch, they will opt for pasta and salad, or cheese, bread and vegetable antipasto for dinner. Bread is never eaten with pasta—for an Italian, that's a no-no! It may be eaten upon finishing the pasta to sop up any leftover sauce.

Assorted vegetables, blanched, steamed or grilled are served firm (*al dente*) at both lunch and dinner. Also offered at the table are extra-virgin olive oil, salt and pepper for seasoning.

The routine of dipping bread into olive oil is not considered an appetizer, but occurs instead during the course of a meal. Eating bread before the meal has a tendency to fill you up and may lessen your enjoyment of the entrée.

Salads in Italy often contain arugula, the green leafy lettuce, with its rich, peppery taste and exceptionally pungent flavor. Arugula is high in folic acid, vitamin A, C and K, iron, calcium and trace minerals. I like to add chopped arugula to pasta or pizza towards the end of the baking period or immediately afterward. This prevents it from wilting from the heat.

Salads piled high with calorically dense toppings like croutons, containing multiple ingredients like in a Cobb salad and served swimming in creamy dressings like Russian, Thousand Island and Ranch are American creations!

MYTHS AND TRUTHS ABOUT ITALIAN FOOD

• *Potatoes, bread, pasta and rice are the most fattening Italian foods.*
  (MYTH)

In the U.S., high-carbohydrate foods like potatoes, bread, pasta and rice have lost their popularity in the past few years, thanks to the Atkins Diet and the gluten-free craze. In fact, there's no proof that high-carbs are more likely to make us gain weight than any other food. Ultimately, it's an excess of calories that piles on the pounds—and it doesn't matter where those extra calories come from!

We know that fat provides twice the amount of calories that carbohydrates do, and it's the fat we add to carbs that increases the calorie content. For example, a three-ounce potato contains 60 calories, and two tablespoons of sour cream adds an additional 60 calories. It's smarter to choose two tablespoons of plain, fat-free yogurt at only 15 calories.

Another culprit is the excessive fat featured in American-style Italian food, like globs of creamy Alfredo sauce served over pasta, or the excess oil, breading and cheese in America's version of Eggplant Parmesan.

Your best choices are minimally processed, high-fiber carbohydrates that fill you up and help promote healthy bowel function. Include more whole cornmeal (used in polenta), whole-wheat pasta and baked or roasted potatoes. Avoid adding fats to these carbohydrate-rich foods. Instead, serve pasta and polenta with a homemade tomato-based sauce and top a potato with fat-free plain yogurt or Dijon mustard. Portion size matters most, so measure one cup of cooked pasta and stick to a three-ounce potato.

• *The Mediterranean diet features heart-healthy olive oil, so olive oil must be safe to indulge in.*
  (MYTH)

63

In 1945, Ancel Keys and other scientists observed that people living in southern Italy were lean and free of heart disease. Their diet consisted of olive oil and an abundance of fruits, vegetables, whole grains, beans, herbs, spices and fish. These people walked an average of nine miles each day! Since then, much has changed in Italy—and throughout the Mediterranean.

While olive oil is high in monounsaturated fats, known to be the healthiest type of fat, it is still 100-percent fat, the most caloric component of food. Since obesity is a risk factor for heart disease, it's best to eat a low-fat diet and use minimally processed (cold-pressed, extra-virgin) olive oil in moderation.

• *Everyone loves pizza, but it's caused a worldwide obesity epidemic.*
  (MYTH)

Americans love pizza almost as much as Italians. Can you imagine dorm life or a Little League team meeting without it? The American pizza has been drastically modified relative to the original Italian version, which came from Naples. It is made with thin flatbread and topped with tomato; the Margherita version has added mozzarella cheese and basil.

Pizza arrived in our country along with the Italian immigrants in the 19th century. Later on, the U.S. food industry commercialized pizza with the emergence of Chicago-style, deep-dish pizza, Pizza Hut pepperoni, and other variations that moved farther away from the original healthy Italian version.

Pizza can definitely fit into a healthy eating plan and contribute many essential nutrients, including calcium, protein and fiber. There are many ways to make a healthy version that will satisfy your taste buds!

When eating out, ask for whole-wheat crust and half the cheese. Top with veggies like artichoke hearts, mushrooms, arugula and peppers instead of pepperoni.

At home, make your own pizza with fresh tomatoes and extra veggies. If you don't have time to make dough from scratch, try whole-grain flatbreads and top with your favorite pizza toppings. Don't forget to end the meal with a large salad drizzled with balsamic vinegar or sprinkled with lemon juice and a touch of olive oil. Italians love to use lemon juice and olive oil with a pinch of salt as a salad dressing. Buon appetito!

PUTTING THE SECRETS OF THE ITALIAN DIET TO WORK FOR YOU

✓ *Favor organically grown and produced food.*

✓ *Include vegetables at every meal. Lowest in calories and highest in nutrients are non-starchy vegetables like salad greens, kale, Swiss chard, artichoke, asparagus, green beans, beets, Brussels sprouts, cabbage, broccoli, cauliflower, carrots, cucumber, eggplant, hearts of palm, leeks, mushrooms, okra, pea pods, peppers, radishes, snap peas, tomato, turnip, jicama, kohlrabi and onion.*

✓ *Learn to count carbs by instinct. Include four to six servings per day (more for those with greater calorie needs). One serving of the following equals 80 to 100 calories: ½ cup cooked pasta, one ounce dry pasta, one slice of bread, a three-ounce potato, ½ cup cooked beans, corn, peas, etc.*

✓ *Never cut your pasta with a knife; instead, roll it neatly around your fork. Make smaller twirls so it will last longer!*

✓ *Eat organic, seasonal fruit when you have a sweet tooth. Include two to four pieces of fruit per day (more for those with greater calorie needs). One serving equals one medium piece of fruit, ½ cup cooked fruit, one cup of berries, etc.*

✓ *Limit fat to cold-pressed, extra-virgin olive oil or high-quality flavored oils in moderation (one to two tablespoons per day).*

✓ *Enjoy mineral water with your meals instead of soft drinks. Reserve cappuccinos and lattes for breakfast only.*

✓ *Consume beans, lentils, peas and unprocessed or dry roasted nuts and seeds instead of animal protein at least three times a week. Avoid nuts and seeds that are roasted in oil or coated with salt.*

✓ *If you are trying to lose weight, use more balsamic vinegar and fresh lemon juice and less olive oil. There are 14 to 20 calories in a tablespoon of balsamic vinegar and four calories in a tablespoon of lemon juice, compared to 120 calories in a tablespoon of olive oil.*

✓ *Reduce balsamic vinegar into sweet syrup on the stovetop: Place vinegar in a small saucepan, then stir and simmer on low heat until the consistency is right. It's delicious over fresh or cooked fruit.*

65

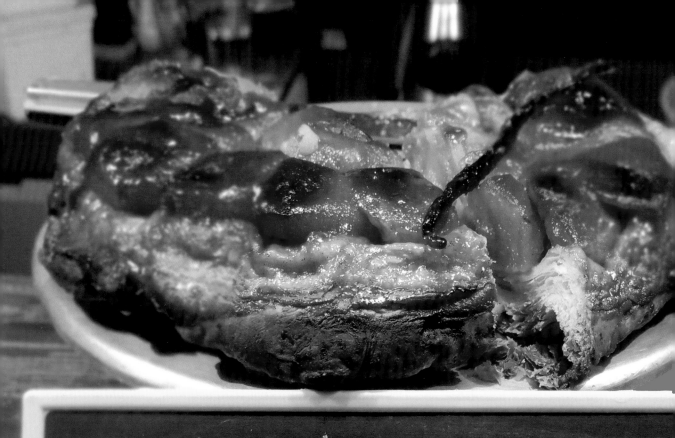

ROSÉ BREAK
5 min.
PLEASE

Chapter 4

THE SECRETS OF THE FRENCH DIET

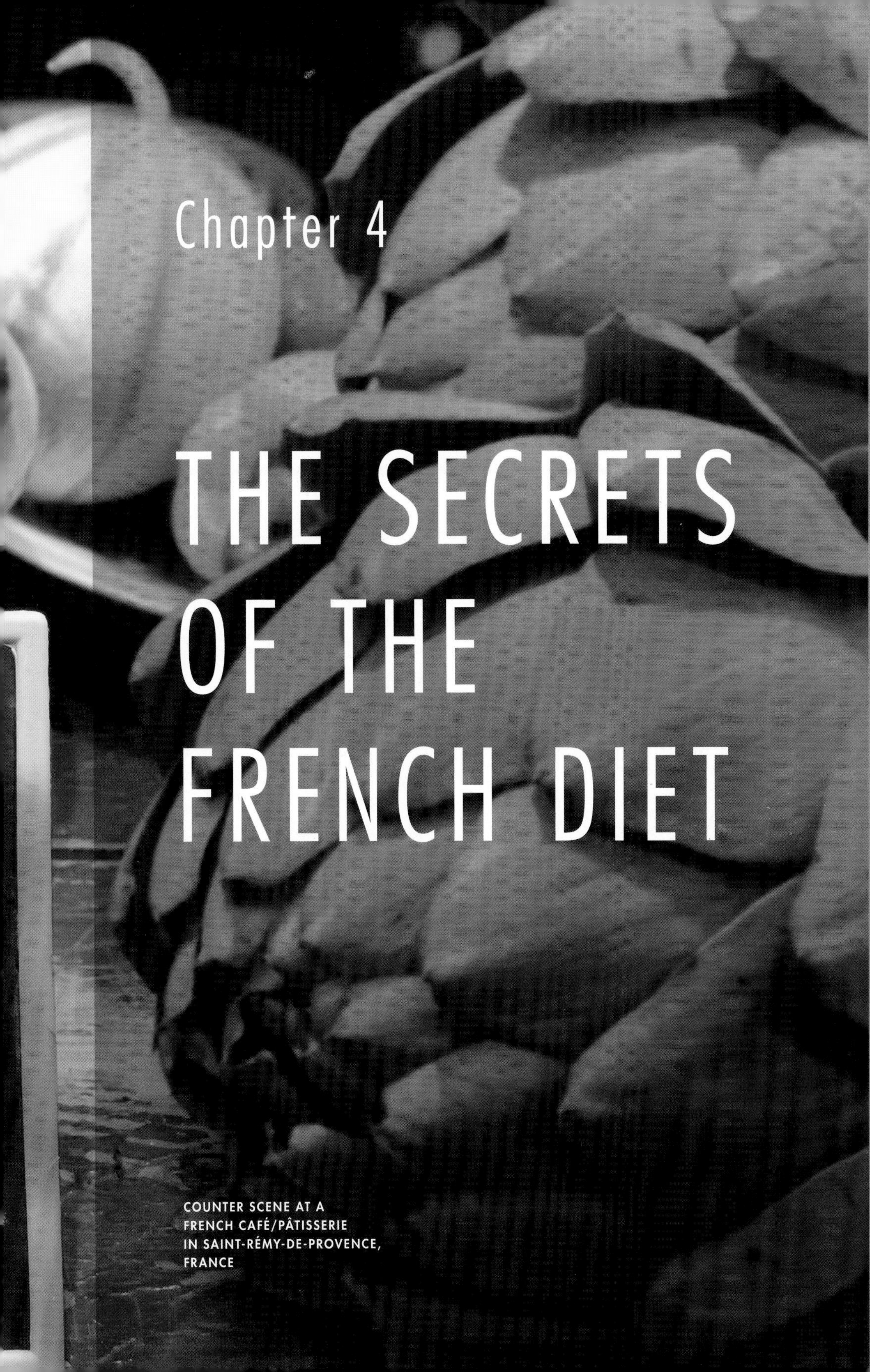

COUNTER SCENE AT A
FRENCH CAFÉ/PÂTISSERIE
IN SAINT-RÉMY-DE-PROVENCE,
FRANCE

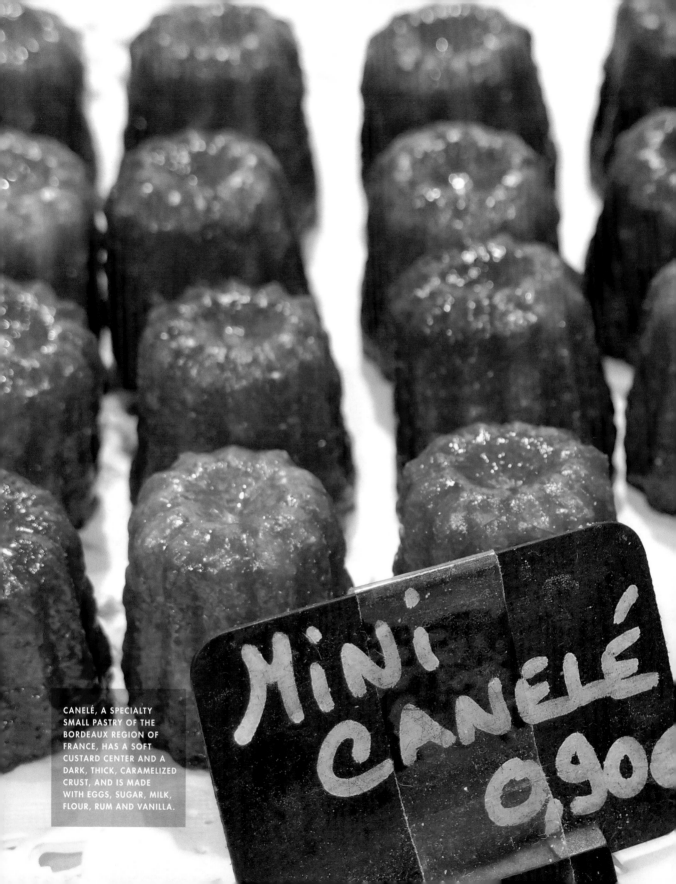

CANELÉ, A SPECIALTY SMALL PASTRY OF THE BORDEAUX REGION OF FRANCE, HAS A SOFT CUSTARD CENTER AND A DARK, THICK, CARAMELIZED CRUST, AND IS MADE WITH EGGS, SUGAR, MILK, FLOUR, RUM AND VANILLA.

MiNi CANELÉ 0,90€

Oh, to be a sophisticated French woman in a sleek pencil skirt, black heels, and a scarf tied just so. These women seem to have it all—a svelte body, the ability to look chic even when toting three small children under the age of five, while enjoying a diet rich in pastries and wine!

Then there is a phenomenon known as the "French Paradox" in which, for some mysterious reason, the French can consume luxurious, fat-laden items like *foie gras* (the fatty liver of a force-fed goose or duck) and rich, creamy sauces like *béarnaise* (made with butter and egg yolks). Yet they have the lowest rate of death from heart disease in Europe. The heart disease death rate in the U.S. is more than 2.5 (2.67 to be precise) times the death rate from heart disease in France. How can this be?

French and American researchers have speculated that perhaps the chemical makeup of wine (red wine, in particular) negated the harmful effects of the fats. In 1991, the TV program, *60 Minutes*, featured an interview with French researcher, Serge Renaud, to discuss this phenomenon. It was the highest rated and most watched television show that week, and viewers were convinced that the answer to the "French Paradox" lay within a bottle of wine.

Once the eager-to-believe American audience accepted that it was okay to eat fatty foods as long as you washed them down with red wine, wine sales skyrocketed! Even the airlines were running out of red wine on domestic flights. Naturally, the U.S. wine industry jumped on the bandwagon and lobbied to add health claims to their wine labels. However, after a protest by the Department of Health and Human Services, the American Medical Association and other consumer advocacy groups, the move was denied.

Red wine became the newest diet fad of the 1990s, matching the oat bran craze of the 1980s. And here is where the Americans and the French differ widely on their approaches to food, and to diet in general. The French are leery of fad diets based on speculative studies and media-hyped messages, and respond to news of this type with a healthy dose of skepticism.

On the other hand, we Americans do not think critically about things we hear and read. We want to believe there is a simple solution to a long-term problem such as obesity, heart disease and diabetes. To get that dose of instant gratification, we'll buy into a quick fix as an easy way out. Instead, we should be doing more research, rather than relying on word of mouth or experts on popular medical TV shows.

The bottom line is, drinking wine with a fatty, cream-based entree is *not* the reason France boasts such impressive health statistics. To find the secret of their health success, I decided to undertake an up-close-and-personal investigation into what Americans could do, like the French, to create a diet of health-boosting foods. I would have to identify foods that could easily be integrated into our lifestyle, resulting in a permanent weight loss and a longer life span.

I first began studying the typical French breakfast, which traditionally begins with a rich, fluffy croissant with a dollop of sweet jam. Sounds indulgent, right? Surprisingly not!

A typical croissant in France weighs slightly more than one ounce and measures 15 inches around, whereas an American croissant weighs almost two ounces and measures 18.5 inches around!

Therefore, a small croissant accompanied by black coffee or coffee with a splash of milk (a typical French breakfast) yields approximately 150 calories and only six grams of fat. The American version is double at 300 calories and 12 grams of fat. So if it's an American-sized croissant you crave, eat half or share it with a friend.

That delicious thin French crêpe with a smear of fruit filling is only 150 calories, while a fried donut oozing with sugary jelly, or an oversized deli muffin, yields 300 to 450 calories. Get the picture? Watch for a yummy crêpe recipe in Part Three.

A traditional "grab and go" French lunch might be a leek quiche or *quiche poireaux* weighing 126 grams, which has 300 calories and 18 grams of fat. Compare this to a fast food cheese pizza that weighs 207 grams and contains 590 calories and 24 grams of fat. A healthy quiche recipe awaits you in Part Three.

A French dinner of salad, veggies, two small lamb chops and a cup of mashed potatoes weighs in at about 500 calories and 18 grams of fat. Compare that to a 16-ounce strip steak and a small portion of fries at 1,300 calories and 78 grams of fat. Oh, my!

Now that France imposes a tax on soft drinks made with either sugars or artificial sweeteners, which came into effect in 2012, there is even more incentive for the French to drink wine!

FRANCE: QUALITY, NOT QUANTITY

To better understand the French diet, you need to understand the importance of food quality and the good agricultural practices of the French. Food is a large contributor to the country's wealth; in fact, France is the only country in Europe completely self-sufficient in food production, offering its citizens high-quality, ecologically friendly products.

France produces grains, sugar beets, flax, potatoes, dairy, pork, poultry, beef and a wide variety of vegetables, fruits and wines. France is also a seafood lover's dream, bordered by the Atlantic Ocean to the north and west, and the Mediterranean Sea to the south.

70

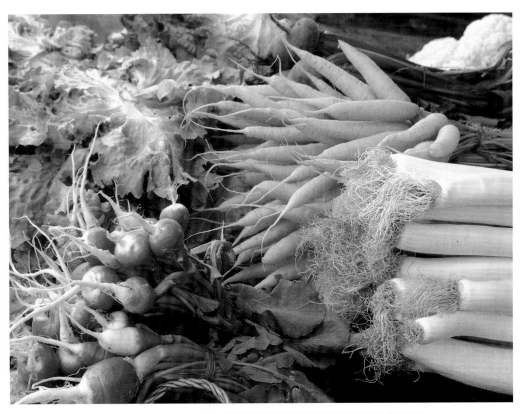

LOCAL VEGETABLES AT A FARMERS MARKET IN DIVONNE-LES-BAINS, FRANCE

The food industry is innovative, modern and competitive, and is one of the largest producers and exporters of food worldwide, known for wines, dairy products, spirits and grains. The best-known vineyards in the world are in Burgundy, Champagne, the Rhône and Loire valleys and Bordeaux.

Since France is the largest country (by land area) in the European Union, the French diet varies widely from north, south, east and west. Climate, cultural differences, available ingredients and regional specialties affect it. The people in the north consume more meat and eat a generally heavier, fattier diet, while southerners in the Mediterranean region eat more fish and vegetables, and enjoy a lighter diet. The north is where the best butter is churned, while the south is famed for its award-winning olive oils.

Compared to other countries, France produces food more naturally, in small batches and with more variety. For example tomatoes are a favorite vegetable in France, and many varieties are produced: ribbed, round, elongated, heirloom, beefsteak, cherry, plum and the list goes on. The quality is so good, you'll rarely bite into one that's less than mouth-watering and delicious!

FRANCE: HOME OF THE GREAT CHEFS

France boasts two of the most renowned culinary cities in the world: Lyon (central-east), the capital of gastronomy, and Paris (northern Île-de-France region). My French language teacher once proclaimed Lyon first and Paris second, as the best food cities in the world.

I spent a lot of time in Lyon with world-class chefs, including Mathieu Viannay, Christian Têtedoie and the one-and-only Paul Bocuse, the most decorated chef in the world and grandfather of *nouvelle cuisine*. He explained that most of France's leading chefs wear a blue-red-and-white-striped collar to identify themselves as *Meilleurs Ouvriers de France* ("Best in Trade of France").

These chefs are awarded the honor of M.O.F. after a rigorous, complicated competition held every four years. If the collar is worn by anyone who is not a M.O.F., he/she can be imprisoned for fraud! This unique system of awards indicates just how serious the French are about food.

Chef Christian Têtedoie says, "French chefs are open to change; we are not snobs as many believe. Even though I only speak French, I travel all over the world to learn from other chefs, and I cooked for the King of Spain last week. I realize that patrons want less

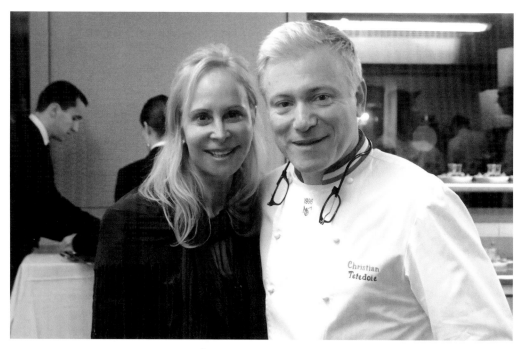

LAYNE AND CHEF CHRISTIAN TÊTEDOIE AT HIS NAMESAKE RESTAURANT IN LYON, FRANCE

complex food and healthier preparations, and I am modifying my cooking techniques. We want our patrons to return often, not just experience our cooking on special occasions. The future promises simple, good ingredients and less complicated preparations. Restaurants here have one seating per meal, while in the U.S., you have three."

"You don't need to go to Marseille for the best bouillabaisse, or to northern France for the best blue lobster. The best ingredients are sent to the cities of Paris and Lyon, since chefs in these cities are willing to pay a premium price for the finest ingredients. The locals get second dibs, because the good stuff is shipped out to Paris and Lyon."

If you visit Lyon, don't leave without dining at the magical and legendary Paul Bocuse restaurant, located just outside the city, which was the inspiration for Disney's movie, "Ratatouille." The movie took place in Paris, but the scenery looks exactly like Paul Bocuse's restaurant in Lyon. Is it a coincidence that Bocuse's son, Jérôme, manages the French pavilion at Walt Disney World's Epcot Center? The Bocuse family has turned out chefs in Lyon dating all the way back to 1765.

In 1965, Paul Bocuse received three Michelin stars, the top award, and has held this ranking longer than anyone else in the world. In 2011, the Culinary Institute of America (CIA) honored Paul Bocuse with the "Chef of the Century" award and named the CIA's French restaurant in Hyde Park, New York, the Bocuse Restaurant.

73

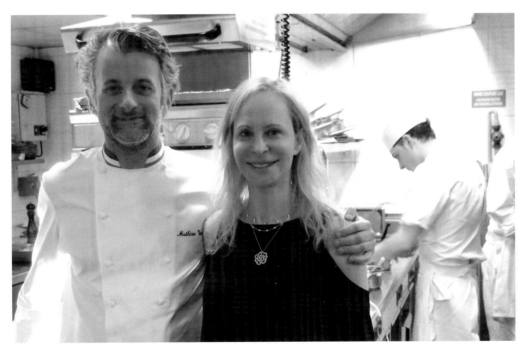

CHEF MATHIEU VIANNAY AND LAYNE IN THE KITCHEN OF LA MÈRE BRAZIER RESTAURANT, LYON, FRANCE

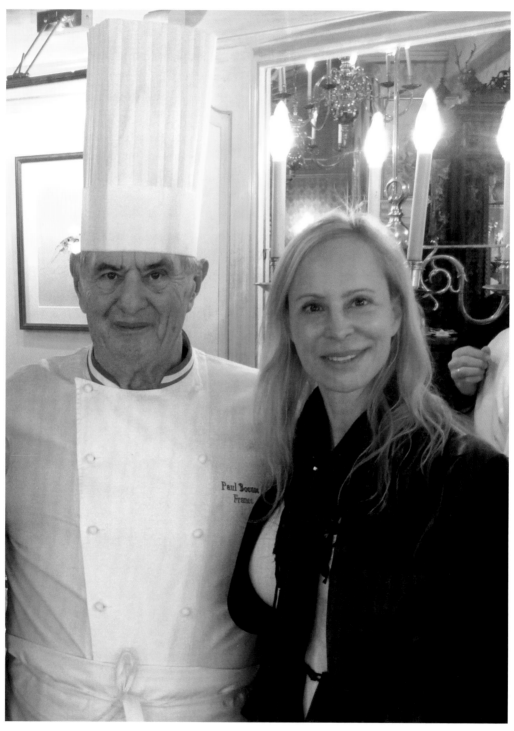

PAUL BOCUSE AND LAYNE AT HIS NAMESAKE RESTAURANT IN LYON, FRANCE

Bocuse started cooking in 1942, and after World War II continued his training at La Mère Brazier, which has remained open since 1933. I mention this restaurant, because it is currently owned and operated by Mathieu Viannay, probably the most innovative, two-star Michelin-rated chef in Lyon today.

On February 11, 2012, I had the pleasure of spending time with Chef Bocuse on his 86th birthday at his restaurant outside Lyon. When I asked him about his diet, he said he was content to dine at home with his family, where he enjoys roasted game with fresh vegetables, bread and wine. Lyon is known for its *bouchons,* a type of casual restaurant that serves traditional Lyonnaise cuisine, with an emphasis on meat dishes.

Paul Bocuse invented *nouvelle cuisine* to lighten up traditional French cooking. At *Les Halles de Lyon or* "The Halls of Food," another Paul Bocuse creation, an amalgam of food vendors and chefs sells a variety of artisanal foods and delicacies. There, I discovered *quenelles,* the torpedo-shaped French dumplings made from flour, milk, eggs and various meats, fish or vegetables. Quenelles are poached in boiling water and then served with a cream sauce. A three-and-a-half-ounce *quenelle* (without sauce) has 170 calories and eight grams of fat.

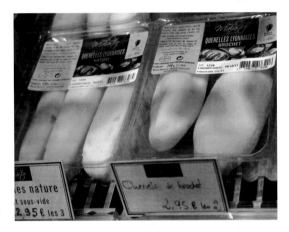

QUENELLES AT THE LES HALLES DE LYON MARKET, FRANCE

75

Whether chatting with chefs or schmoozing with locals, I discovered that the food culture in France is revered, offering a strong foundation for a sophisticated approach to life. It is a quality that makes the French so fascinating to everyone else in the world.

LAYNE'S FRENCH FAVORITES

My favorite French cuisine is native rural or peasant-style food, which is simpler than their urban fare. Historically, this is because fruits, vegetables and grains were cheap and local. Peasant foods are dishes that can be made in one pot or pan, like *Socca de Nice* (chickpea patty), *coq au vin* (chicken braised in wine), and *pistou* (a French version of pesto made with basil, garlic and olive oil).

On the other hand, in the fancy restaurants of France and America, the wealthier classes historically consumed a high-quality meal or *haute cuisine*—with dishes containing complex, creamy sauces, cheeses, pâtés and pastries. All served with fine wine, of course! However, whether meals are peasant or "high" cuisine, both French versions trump America's fast food nation nutritionally.

My favorite dishes are *ratatouille*, a stew made with tomatoes, eggplant, sweet peppers and herbs (recipe in Part Three) and *bouillabaisse*, a hearty soup made with at least three kinds of fish in a broth of onions, tomatoes, saffron and herbs such as bay leaf, sage and thyme. Both dishes are nutritious, low fat and satisfying.

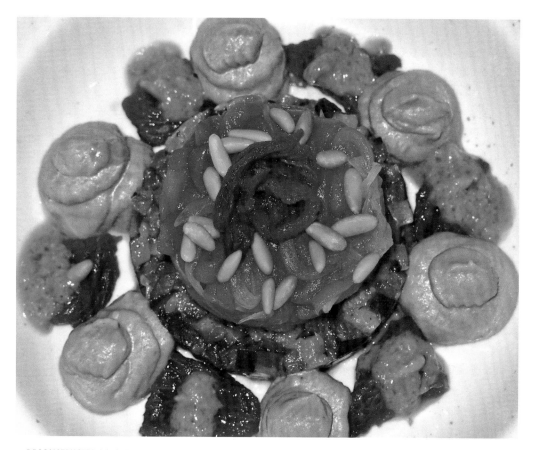

DECONSTRUCTED RATATOUILLE BY CHEF CHRISTIAN ETIENNE AT HIS NAMESAKE RESTAURANT IN AVIGNON, FRANCE

In Avignon, a city of Provence, I enjoyed a memorable meal by Chef Christian Etienne, in celebration of the local tomato harvest. He prepared a "deconstructed ratatouille," where each ingredient was prepared individually and presented in a different way on one plate. It was a medley of local vegetables, including purees of eggplant and zucchini, slivers of red peppers, pine nuts and roasted heirloom tomatoes. I often relish the tastes of Provence's summertime harvest, including fresh herbs, which made his creation the perfect ratatouille!

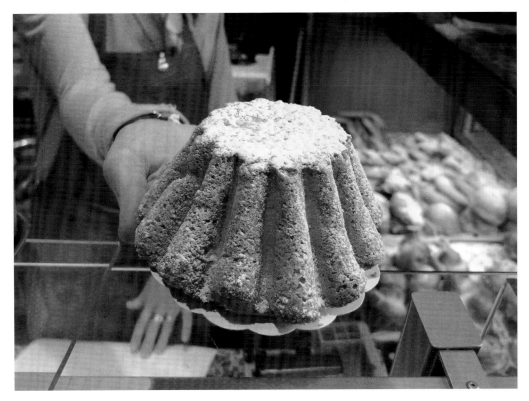

VERITABLE BISCUIT DE SAVOIE AT BOULANGERIE ARTISANALE IN ANNECY, FRANCE

My favorite cake is the French version of a sponge cake called *Veritable Biscuit de Savoie* from Annecy, a town in the Savoie region an hour outside of Geneva, Switzerland. It is made with flour, cornstarch, eggs, sugar and vanilla, with no additional fats. The texture is light, yet it has a rich, satisfying flavor, because only the freshest ingredients are used.

It is not as sweet and heavy as sponge cake. One average slice of sponge cake is 220 calories and has 15 grams of fat, compared to this regional version containing only 148 calories and 2.7 grams of fat.

In the French Basque region (southwest), on the sandy beaches of Biarritz and Saint-Jean-de-Luz, there is an influence by the great chefs of the Spanish Basque. Here, I discovered the Espelette pepper, a spicy, yet sweet red chili pepper named for the town where it's grown. *Pipérade* is a specialty dish of this region and is made with Espelette pepper, onion, tomato and egg. You'll find a tasty *Pipérade* recipe in Part Three.

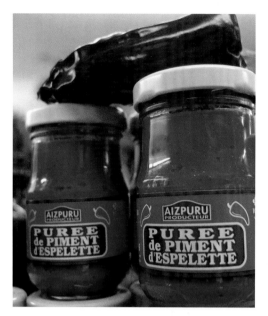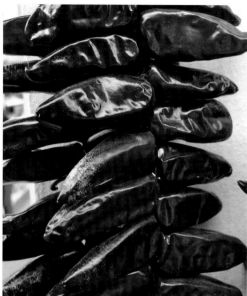

ESPELETTE PEPPER (GROUND AND DRIED) AT A SHOP IN BIARRITZ, FRANCE

The cuisine of southeast France (Provence, French Riviera and the island of Corsica) is centered on local farmers markets and fresh seafood. Some of my favorites during spring and summer harvest include figs, tomatoes, eggplant, zucchini, peppers, radishes, asparagus, rice, olives and herbs. These foods are best paired with a refreshing, local rosé wine to complement meals from the area.

FRENCH DIETARY GUIDELINES

I was delighted to discover that France's National Institute for Prevention and Health Education offers the most creative and enjoyable food guides I'd ever seen! They have designed 25 individual guides under the title, "The Food Guide For All" (*Le Guide Alimentaire Pour Tous, 2002*).

Each guide is based on a person's personality, habits and lifestyle. There are guides for everyone—those who are health-conscious, those who are casual about what they eat, those who prepare family meals, those who are poor, those who eat out a lot, those who skip meals, etc.

On the cover of every guide is a "portrait"—an image of a happy face constructed out of foods representing that person's nutritional type. The portraits are billed as "nutrition recommendations," though they are more artistic than information-based.

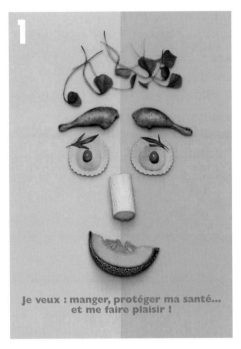

Je veux : manger, protéger ma santé... et me faire plaisir !

I WANT TO: EAT, PROTECT MY HEALTH AND MAKE ME HAPPY

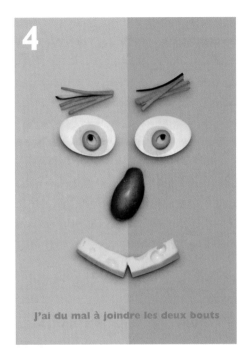

J'ai du mal à joindre les deux bouts

I FIND IT HARD TO MAKE ENDS MEET

There are so many styles of eating that one size cannot fit all, hence the whimsical 25 food faces. France's overall health and nutrition messages are *eat well, stay active and protect your health.* The French are advised to limit fat, salt and sugar, drink more water, exercise daily, eat less animal protein, and eat more fruits, vegetables, whole grains, potatoes and legumes. Alcohol consumption should not exceed the equivalent of two glasses of wine per day for women and three for men. Physical activity should include at least one-half hour of brisk walking per day to get just enough vitamin D from sunlight.

The French enjoy an active family lifestyle; they walk often, ski, swim, bicycle and play sports. While gyms are less popular with women than here in the United States, French women do enjoy Pilates, a method of stretching, strengthening and toning muscles. Yoga is also becoming more popular. The French drink more sparkling water than soda, and enjoy both coffee and herbal tea. The world-famous Evian water is found in Evian, France, close to Geneva, Switzerland.

The French limit fat, sugar and salt by eating a diet of unprocessed foods. They prefer natural and local foods, enjoying legumes such as beans and lentils as much as animal proteins. Seasonal fruits and vegetables are staples of their daily diet, along with a fresh *baguette* (thin loaf of bread).

WHAT *ABOUT* THE FRENCH PARADOX?

One theory to explain France's lower rate of heart disease is the presence of resveratrol, an antioxidant found in red wine. However, you would have to drink one thousand bottles of red wine a day to obtain the equivalent amounts that are now being used in health studies—and that would be toxic to your liver! Resveratrol is also found in the skins of cranberries, blueberries, grapes and pomegranate seeds. Research is now being conducted to find out if this antioxidant, when administered in large doses, can indeed prolong life and improve health.

In my opinion, the French Paradox has more to do with the difference in our core values regarding food. The French aim for quality over quantity, reflecting pride in their products, and the best quality ingredients are available for everyone. Instead of being addicted to fast foods, the French focus on well-prepared foods made from fresh ingredients.

To satisfy their sweet cravings, the French might choose a square of chocolate at 27 calories and two grams of fat, rather than a quart of ice cream at 2,000 calories and 128 grams of fat.

Best of all, the French are masters at exercising portion control, which is one reason why they are slimmer and healthier than we Americans.

Now, let's take a closer look at their diet!

THE HEALTHY FRENCH DIET

No matter where you are in France, food is not just something you pick up at the supermarket. The French choose each of their foods carefully, according to its qualities and origins. While fine sauces and elaborate desserts are easily available, especially in larger towns and cities, daily fare is much simpler and more wholesome.

It is not always easy to find a wide range of international cuisine in France, and searching for an Indian or Mexican restaurant can require long-distance travel. On the other hand, Moroccan couscous is the most widely eaten staple in France, and Italian pasta is also popular. At home, the French prefer using foods that are both diverse and quick to prepare. Available regional produce will heavily influence "what's cooking" in the kitchen, with fresh vegetables and fruits appearing regularly at every meal.

To us Americans, it seems as if the French eat small portions, but in reality they eat "normal" portions of a predominantly natural-foods diet. In comparison, we have fallen victim to supersized portions and trend toward convenience and processed foods. And while it may seem as if the French eat more saturated fat (butter, cream and foie gras), they actually eat moderate amounts of fat (due to smaller portions) and balance it with fresh vegetables, fruits, grains and legumes.

The French love lentils, beets and figs as much as they love cheese, lamb and pork—you just don't read about it. And the high-fat foods that the French eat provide nutrition, unlike the poor nutritional, processed foods of the American diet. The French would rather pay more for quality food than waste money on junk food.

The French eat until they feel satisfied and full, whereas Americans eat until their oversized plates are empty or until everyone else is done eating! One explanation is that the French were not subject to "The Clean Plate Club" campaign, which was introduced by the U.S. federal government in 1917 during World War I to encourage families to finish their entire meal. It was reinstated in 1947 after the Great Depression and World War II. Unfortunately, this practice of "cleaning our plates" has become

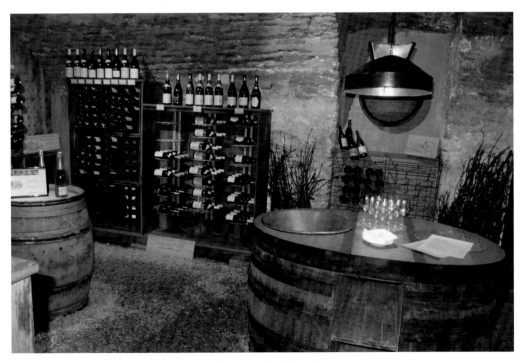

LE CAVE À VINS (WINE CAVE) IN BURGUNDY, FRANCE

a carry-over habit to the current-day American lifestyle. Instead of relying on our internal cues of hunger, we practice habits that no longer serve us. Compounded with supersized portions, we consume way too many calories than what is needed for a slim and healthy body.

Now, let's take a closer look at some of the traditional and regional foods in France that are eaten *in moderation* by the French.

The southwest is known for food prepared with duck, prunes, oysters, mushrooms and truffles (underground mushrooms) with, of course, a full-bodied red Bordeaux wine to go with it.

Normandy in the northwest is best known for its apples (used for cider and the famed Calvados-apple brandy), Camembert cheese and its seafood from the Atlantic Ocean, especially mussels, blue lobster and oysters.

Next door, in Brittany, you can't escape the crêpe, commonly eaten sweet rather than savory.

The staples of the northeast are my favorite winter vegetables—beets, potatoes and cabbage. *Charcuterie* or cold, cooked, salted and dried meats, similar to our deli meats are thinly sliced, savored and eaten in small quantities. Examples are ham, bacon and sausage. This region is most famous for champagne.

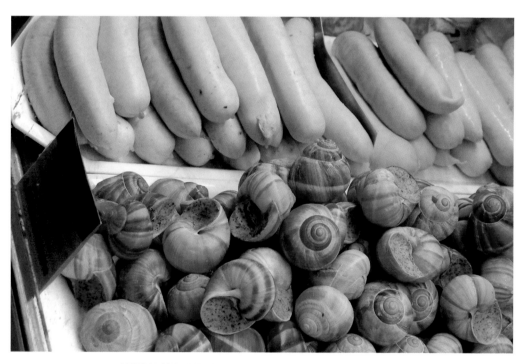

SAUSAGE AND ESCARGOT AT LES HALLES DE LYON MARKET, FRANCE

The eastern region is heavily influenced by German food, like pickled cabbage and pork. Savory foods like *Quiche Lorraine* originated in this area. Other popular foods include jams and preserves. Burgundy, in the central eastern region, is famous for Burgundy wine—think *boeuf bourguignon* (beef burgundy) and *coq au vin* (chicken baked in wine). Dijon mustard and snails *(escargots)* also originated in this area.

FOOD SHOPPING, FRENCH STYLE

The French shop for food in the charming, proprietor-owned shops of butchers or *boucheries*, fishmongers or *poissoneries*, greengrocers or *marchand de fruits et de legumes*, cheesemakers or *magasins fromage*, pastry bakers or *patisseries*, and bread bakers or *boulangeries*. You'll find pastry and bread shops everywhere!

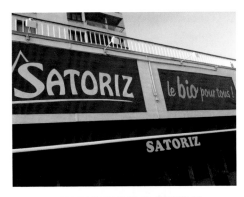

SATORIZ NATURAL FOOD MARKET IN
FERNEY VOLTAIRE, FRANCE

By law, bakeries in France must mix, knead, leaven, and bake their own bread on premises without ever being frozen. Preservatives are not allowed to be used in any bread.

When I lived in Europe, like the French, I began to bring home the freshest foods from the farmers markets, occasionally finishing at the Carrefour supermarket, or *supermarché*, the largest retail chain in France. The truth about France is that you can choose to eat "old school," or go as packaged and convenient as you desire. However, even in these modern times, most French choose the "old school" ways.

I often skipped over the border from Switzerland to France to shop in Satoriz, a chain of 83 organic markets throughout France. One week, they had a local variety of white carrots.

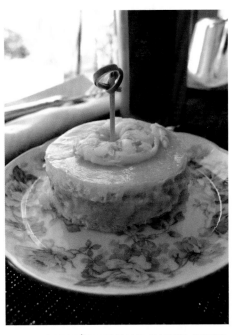

SANDWICH AT HÔTEL DU PALAIS, BIARRITZ, FRANCE

Did you know that carrots are the second most popular vegetable in the world, with potatoes number one? When U.S. cooks tried to re-introduce the purple carrot, another ancient variety, they were disturbed to see that other ingredients in the pan absorbed the purple color. They soon stopped including these unique carrots in their meals.

Tea rooms, or *salons de thé,* are found throughout France. They have longer opening hours than restaurants and serve tea, coffee, pastries, cakes, sandwiches and sometimes salads. You'll also find these in the French regions of Switzerland.

SPECIALTY FOODS, FRENCH-STYLE

There are three staples of the French diet that you'll find in every part of France: bread, cheese and wine! This combo makes a great meal by itself. Just add some crudité (assorted raw or slightly steamed cut-up veggies), and you'll be all set!

A baguette is a long, skinny loaf of crusty bread, which according to French law must follow a recipe of essentially wheat flour, water, salt and yeast. If you arrive in Paris and don't see a person with a baguette tucked into a bag, you can be pretty sure that the end of the world has officially arrived. A baguette is a regular feature of most French meals and can be sliced or torn apart by hand to accompany the entrée at any meal. It can also be cut in half to make sandwiches. Both here and in France, you'll find that the usual white bread version is also made with whole-grains, which are higher in fiber and nutrients.

While there is a best baguette competition every year, according to a recent *New York Times* article, the average Frenchman eats half a baguette a day, compared to almost a whole one in 1970. Women eat about one-third less than men. The demise may be linked to less artisan bakers making crusty, handmade breads. Or maybe the French are opting for other types of bread like *pain complet* (whole-wheat) or *céréales* (multi-grain).

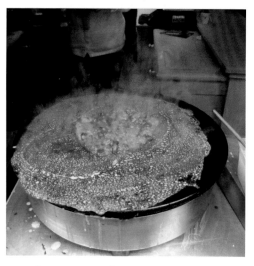

CRÊPERIE IN SAINT-RÉMY-DE-PROVENCE, FRANCE

Crêpes, very thin pancakes, are made from a simple batter of egg, flour, milk and a small amount of oil or butter; and salt. A crêpe can be topped with a variety of ingredients, such as a sweet version stuffed with bananas and strawberries, or savory style filled with chicken and hearts, among many hundreds of possible combinations. Crêpes are perfect at breakfast, lunch, snack, dinner or dessert. They are very easy to make at home using a crêpe pan. Alternatively, there are natural, packaged mixes or imported, pre-made crêpes, found in the produce section. One seven-inch crêpe averages 110 calories and five grams of fat. A crêpe recipe can be found in Part Three.

Some of the most famous cheeses (*les fromages*) in the world are from France and include:

Brie, a creamy, rich, yet mild cow's milk cheese, is produced with a white, edible rind of mold. It is named after the area in which it is produced, which is not far from Paris. One ounce averages 95 calories and eight grams of fat and is a good source of protein and B vitamins.

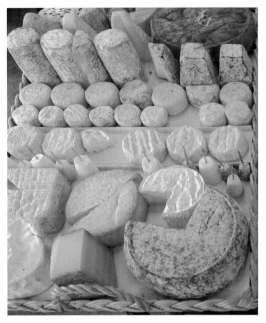

CHEESE BASKET AT PAUL BOCUSE RESTAURANT IN LYON, FRANCE

Camembert, similar to Brie but slightly stronger, is almost always eaten with a baguette and is one of the most popular foods in France. One ounce averages 85 calories and seven grams of fat.

Roquefort, a sheep's-milk blue cheese, is one of France's most famous cheeses and one of the oldest. Crumbly and tangy, one ounce averages 105 calories and nine grams of fat and is high in calcium and protein.

Fromage blanc is a "fresh cheese" that is creamy and soft and made from whole or skim milk. One ounce of the skim milk version averages 15 calories and zero grams of fat and is very high in calcium. Sometimes cream is added, which raises the calories and fat. It is served sweet with fruit or savory like cream cheese.

Cheeses are broadly divided into two categories: fresh (unripened) and aged (ripened). Cheese is made from either cow's milk, sheep's milk or goat's milk.

Ripened and aged cheeses are so flavorful that the French enjoy just a sliver with fresh fruit at the end of a meal. For them, this *is* dessert! Stick to a one-ounce serving.

It looks like a one-inch square cube. Fresh cheeses like fromage blanc are naturally lower in calories, sodium and fat.

Olive oils from Provence are as complex and prized as the finest French wines. In fact, there would be no local cuisine without the fruits of the olive trees. The olive oils from the fertile soil and microclimates of Provence range from peppery, earthy and fruity to robust, moderate and mild. It is sheer delight to dip a piece of crusty French bread into olive oil produced in Provence.

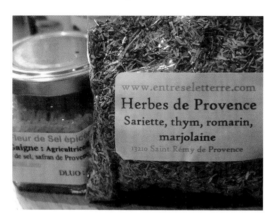

HERBES DE PROVENCE FROM PROVENCE, FRANCE

Herbes de Provence is the famous blend of dried herbs from this area. Besides its herbs, Provence is known for its lavender fields, abundant fruits and vegetables, olive oils and rosé wines. Herbes de Provence typically includes savory, rosemary and thyme. In the U.S., the name is used generically, and there is no guarantee that an herb blend so named is actually from Provence.

Blue Lobster or *Homard Bleu* from the northwest coast of France is far more flavorful than other lobsters, and if you love lobster, you must try it at least once in your life. While dining at a fine restaurant in France, my husband ordered a first course of lobster salad. Knowing that European lobsters are smaller, we were surprised when the dish appeared with quite a large lobster. I asked the waiter why this was so, and he replied (in French), "We import Maine lobsters, because the tourists are dissatisfied with the local small lobsters from France. And besides, Maine lobsters are cheaper!"

Black figs from France are the most addictive fruit in the world. (Maybe that's why they are considered aphrodisiacs.) They are grown in a controlled region of Provence that guarantees high-production standards, so these figs are a perfect balance of firmness with a sweet, strawberry jam-like pulp. The flavor can have a hint of rhubarb or watermelon and goes perfectly with cheese as a dessert. They can complement any meal with poultry or meat dishes as well.

California produces black figs from late June through early fall. My favorite way to prepare fresh figs is by halving them, drizzling them with balsamic vinegar and roasting them in the oven. (See recipe in Chapter 14.) I cook with dried figs in the winter, roasting them with poultry or dicing them with cooked grains.

A TYPICAL DAY OF BLISSFUL EATING FOR THE FRENCH

Back in the times of the Versailles kings, their great feasts typified the passion of the French for the highest quality food and their desire to create ever-more-impressive *"pièces de résistance."* An egg, for example, could be boiled or poached, fried or scrambled and placed on a piece of bread, or it could be turned into a fluffy omelet, a dense quiche, or a velvety hollandaise sauce. Even today, the French can eat with simplicity or decadence, but always with an innate sense of how to balance both.

For breakfast *(le petit déjeuner),* the French will eat a version of bread or pastry, such as a croissant, *pain au chocolat* (chocolate-filled roll or croissant), or *tartine* (an open-faced sandwich with jam or cheese), or perhaps yogurt with a piece of fruit. Coffee, usually espresso or *café au lait* (coffee with milk) is a favorite beverage of the French. They tend to prefer tea late in the afternoon to wind down from the day.

Like the Swiss, the French choose to eat larger meals at lunch *(le déjeuner),* rather than a rushed version at the office. Lunch out can either be a two-hour, multi-course meal, a relaxed lunch at home, or a simple salad or sandwich from a street vendor or sandwich shop. Vegetarian options are more common in France than in Switzerland.

When dining out for lunch, the French begin with a starter called *l'entrée.* Note that in America, "entrée" refers to the main course, but in France, it indicates a first course. The *entrée* is more substantial than *hors d'œuvres.* It is more like a half-size version of a main course, and could be a soup, salad, *pâté, quenelle,* etc. The main course, or *plat principal,* is a meat, poultry or fish and typically includes a starch and vegetable. A dessert and/or fruit and cheese follow. Lunch is often accompanied by wine.

More casual restaurants will serve crêpes, salads and omelets. *Salad Niçoise,* originally from the city of Nice in the south of France, is a popular main course—a large mixed salad of lettuce, tomatoes, green beans, tuna, eggs, anchovies and olives tossed with a light coating of vinaigrette dressing.

An afternoon snack, or *le goûter,* is sometimes enjoyed on the way home from work or school. It might be a small *baguette* sandwich or a *quiche* from a street vendor or at the train station. Interestingly, adults do not snack often in France, and children only snack once a day, in the afternoon. American kids, on the other hand, tend to snack more often, often due to boredom or while watching television.

Tchin-tchin (cheers!) leads to the traditional pre-dinner *l'aperitif,* a French social habit where drinks are made from local alcohols and served with appetizers or light snacks, known as *hors d'œuvres,* like olives, tapenade and nuts. Consider adding a flute of champagne or a *kir* cocktail made with *crème de cassis* or black currant liqueur mixed with white wine.

Dinner, or *le diner,* depends on whether you had a big lunch or a modest one. Generally, multi-course dinners are reserved for special occasions. Bread, salad, a meat course and a dessert (often fruit and/or cheese) will typically comprise the meal. If meat is eaten for lunch, dinner might be soup, salad, eggs, yogurt, bread and fruit. Another dinner might be pasta or couscous with vegetables.

Because school lunches in France are often elaborate, they can include mussels, roasted guinea fowl and steamed artichokes. Therefore, parents opt for a lighter approach to dinner, such as pasta with cheese and salad. On special occasions, dinners feature more courses, and the dinner table is set as fashionably as the French themselves are dressed!

Interestingly, fast food is available in France, but unlike in the U.S., McDonald's in Paris is busiest during the Parisians set meal times of 12 noon to 2 p.m., and 7 p.m. to 9 p.m. Also, there is a rumor that McDonald's will be introducing waiter service in some outlets in Paris, so that "fast" food might actually be a slower, healthier and more French affair.

Are you wondering about dessert? For evenings out and special occasions, the French enjoy a sliver or two of cheese (no more than three slivers) and one or two *petits fours,* those bite-size delicious confections. Alternatively, fruit-based desserts like poached

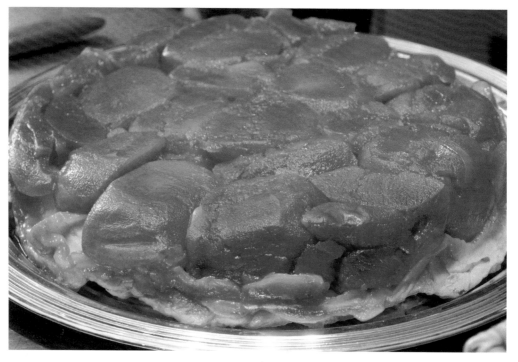

APPLE TART AT I FEEL BIO CAFÉ IN GENEVA, SWITZERLAND

pears, fruit-filled meringue and fruit tarts are favored. At home they are content with yogurt and fresh fruit.

We cannot leave this chapter without mentioning *mousse au chocolat,* since everyone knows this famous French food. I make a light version in the blender with tofu, cocoa powder, blackstrap molasses and maple syrup. (See recipe in Chapter 14.)

Speaking of chocolate, if you should come across Richart chocolate from Lyon, (sold at *les Halles de Lyon)*, available in the U.S. and online, try it. It's been called "the best special occasion chocolate" since 1925.

The French traditionally end a meal with coffee or tea, commonly a *tisane* (herbal tea) and a liqueur, considered a *digestif.* The word *liqueur* is derived from the Latin word, *liquifacere,* which means "to dissolve." The French believe that digestion is aided when you drink a small quantity of Cognac, Armagnac, Calvados or Eau de Vie (clear fruit brandy).

I learned quite a few table-manner tips in France. These include: keep your hands in sight at all times and don't fold them in your lap; never take a bite from a whole piece of bread—instead, tear off a small piece; and show your waiter that you are finished eating by neatly placing your knife and fork (with tines down) on the right side of the dish. Young children learn these rules of etiquette when very young, at home as well as in the classroom. The French like to eat at home more often than in a restaurant.

Good table manners, when practiced diligently tend to slow down the pace of eating, which is good for digestion and helps the brain register fullness.

MYTHS AND TRUTHS ABOUT FRENCH FOOD

• *The French don't differentiate between good fats and bad fats.*
  (TRUTH)

The French eat meat, cheese and butter. They also eat fruit, vegetables and grains. Our beloved American chef, Julia Child, who helped bring French food to an American audience, said: "I think one of the terrible things today is that people have this deathly fear of food: fear of eggs, say, or fear of butter. Most doctors feel that you can have a little bit of everything."

She also said something that I heard time and again in France: "Fat gives food flavor." Indeed, Julia lived to be 91 years old and was producing cooking shows and cookbooks until the end of her life.

This offers us a profound lesson. Instead of eating rich food under the cover of darkness at home, enjoy it openly with your friends. You may really want that piece of steak for dinner, but instead, you order a salad and think of nothing but the steak! Then, to satisfy your frustrated taste buds, you allow yourself a candy bar on the way home. Wouldn't it have been better to share a steak with a friend, as well as the salad? That way, you would have had the best of both worlds, and perhaps wouldn't have needed that overprocessed (high in trans fats) snack on the way home.

Like the French, choose quality foods. You are responsible for the right balance and proper portions of food on your plate! Chapter 6 will explain this. And remember that an occasional indulgence is okay. Because American portion sizes are larger than those of the French, you can share, eat half and take the rest home, or order a smaller portion.

- *Wine is a staple of the French diet, but not a cure-all.*
  (TRUTH)

France is probably more famous for its wines than any other country in the world. There has been a marked fall in the production of *vin ordinaire,* or table wine, because the EEC (European Economic Community) policy now favors an increase in the output of more expensive, high-quality wines.

This may be why French consumption of wine has actually been cut in half since the 1960s, when the average person drank 160 liters per year (or 676 cups). According to the French Ministry of Agriculture, it's now down to only 57 liters per year (or 241 cups). The French are opting for quality over quantity, drinking in moderation, and saving their wine indulgences for the weekends or social occasions.

Studies have shown that drinking a moderate amount of any type of alcohol may aid in preventing heart disease by raising your good cholesterol (HDL).

- *The French are very involved with their food.*
  (TRUTH)

Most French people are fascinated with where their food is coming from, how it's grown or raised, how it's prepared, where the best places are to get the best products, etc. They often consume multi-course meals, as is true in much of Europe. In the U.S., we also eat multi-course meals, except each course is double or triple the size of the European portion size.

The French favor farmers markets that provide fresh seasonal produce and foods made in small batches. We favor big-box stores like Wal-Mart and Costco that sell quantity at discounts. The French tend to shop several times a week, preparing their meals around the freshest available foods. We prefer to shop once a week, with the expectation that the food we buy will last for one week or longer.

• *The French eat multiple courses, but they are always small servings.*
  (MYTH)

The French eat normal-sized portions. We Americans eat supersized portions, so in comparison to what we are used to, French food quantities look small.

Remember the croissant I mentioned at the beginning of the chapter? The French portion size was one ounce! Why aren't the French hungry when they eat so much less than we do? Fortunately for them, their tummies have been trained to expect the right amount. The result: trimmer, healthier bodies.

In contrast, we Americans have had our stomachs stretched by supersized portions, and when the stomach gets used to accommodating that much food, it rebels when we try to cut back. Happily, this trend can be reversed, and I'll get to it in Part Two.

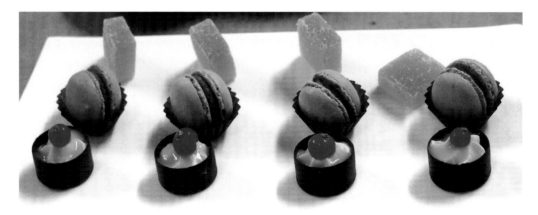

PETITS FOURS AT L'HOSTELLERIE DE LEVERNOIS IN BURGUNDY, FRANCE

The French eat normal portions more slowly. As they eat, they cut their food into smaller and smaller pieces, making the food last longer. When they eat dessert, they don't sit down to a big hunk of cake. Instead, they'll eat a *petit four*, which means "small oven" and is a bite-size fancy cake, cookie, or confection that's tempting both visually and gastronomically. Best of all, it's just enough to satisfy your sweet tooth. An average *petit four* weighs 15 grams and has 60 calories and 1.75 grams of fat.

The French typically use daintier utensils and smaller plates, cups and drinking glasses. Our dishes in the 1970s only averaged nine inches, which Europeans now typically use at home, but today, American plates average 12 inches. Larger plates make a serving of food appear smaller and can deceive us as to how much food we're actually eating.

In an experiment, scientists gave children at camp larger cereal bowls (14.7 inches in diameter) than usual. Not surprisingly, they consumed significantly more cereal compared to those given normal-size bowls (eight-and-a-half inches in diameter). Yet they thought they were eating less than the campers eating from the normal-sized cereal bowls because larger dishes tempt us to put more food on them, while tricking us into thinking we've eaten less.

You can, however, use portion control to your advantage. Later, in Part Two, you'll learn how to trick yourself into eating more veggies and fewer sweet desserts.

- *The French don't often go to gyms.*
  (TRUTH)

You're not likely to find many men and women jogging along the streets of Paris, nor are the airwaves cluttered with ads for reduced monthly fees to the gym. The French generally dislike gyms; to them, it's a waste of their time that could be better spent in good conversation with their friends.

Instead, France is a nation of strollers. Men and women can be seen walking together for miles, chatting and enjoying the view. And while they do love such sports as tennis, swimming and skiing, they reject the "no pain, no gain" approach. Instead, they walk a lot and keep moving throughout the day.

- *The French like steak (but not a 24-ounce size).*
  (TRUTH)

French beef and American beef taste different. French cattle are primarily grass-fed, as opposed to American corn- and feedlot-fed cattle. That's why the meat in France is less marbled, leaner and tougher than American beef—so don't overcook it!

What we can learn from the French is that it's possible to eat red meat in moderation. True, it's not necessarily good for your heart or your colon, but if you stick to a reasonable quantity, such as a three- to six-ounce cooked portion as part of a balanced diet, you can add it to your eating plan. Whether you prefer pork, lamb or beef, eat it like the French and choose leaner cuts, buy from sources that sell organic and grass-fed or pasture-raised varieties, trim away visible fat, and use cooking methods that don't require adding extra fat.

PUTTING THE SECRETS OF THE FRENCH DIET TO WORK FOR YOU

✓ *There are no forbidden foods, as long as you eat a balanced diet in the right portions.*

✓ *Linger over lunch with friends rather than dining at your computer.*

✓ *Eat mindfully, and consciously choose higher-quality ingredients.*

✓ *Dine when you are hungry, not when habit tells you to do so. Europeans eat dinner at a later hour than most Americans, because that's when they feel hungry.*

✓ *On special occasions, share a dessert four ways, to keep in line with the size of petits fours. To end a meal, opt for low-fat yogurt and fruit. Keep high-fat cakes, cookies and chips out of the house (out of sight, out of mind), but do keep a fruit bowl in your fridge.*

✓ *Train your eyes to recognize a healthy-size portion of food. A portion of meat, poultry or fish is three to six ounces cooked (depending upon how many calories you need per day). A satisfying portion of pasta is one cup cooked. You may want to begin weighing and measuring foods to get the hang of it. (See Appendix for What Counts as One Serving.)*

✓ *Remember, the French don't eat small portions; we Americans eat supersized portions. Eat until you feel satisfied and full, rather than eating until your oversized plate is empty or until everyone else is done eating! In other words, get in touch with your own sense of fullness rather than relying on external cues.*

✓ *If you have not been advised otherwise by your physician or health professional, drink wine moderately and with meals. For weight control, don't exceed more than 16 ounces per week. White wine served chilled goes well with seafood and vegetarian dishes. Red wine served at room temperature is a good match for red meat dishes, but don't be afraid to drink some with salmon and other hearty fish and poultry dishes.*

✓ *If you are sensitive to the sulfites in wine, try organically produced wine with no added sulfites. Sulfites are naturally occurring in wine, so wine cannot be 100-percent sulfite-free. See the Appendix for definitions of organic (there are two types), biodynamic and sustainable wine.*

93

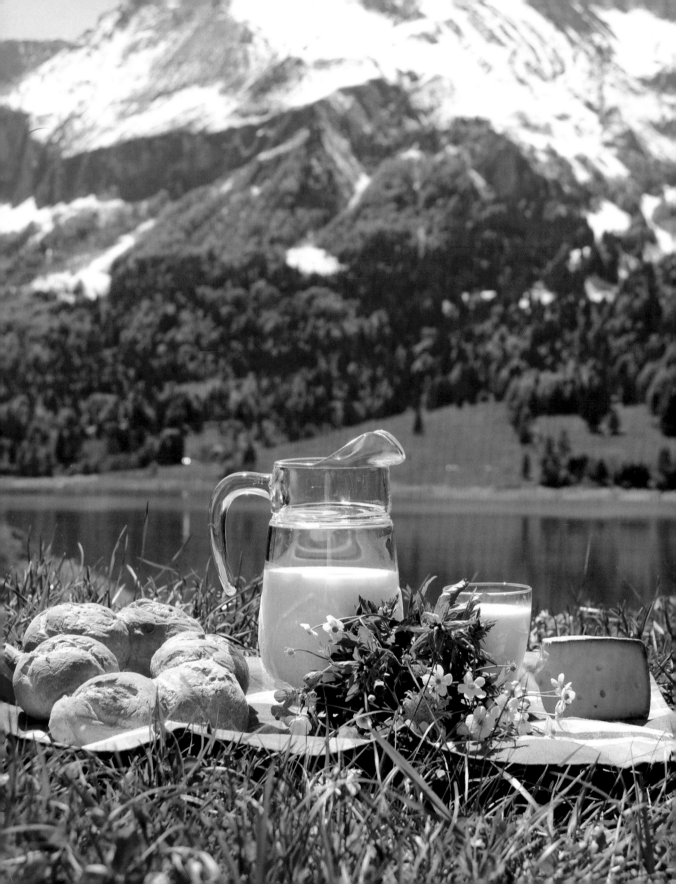

Part Two

GOING BEYOND THE MEDITERRANEAN DIET

PICNIC OF MILK, CHEESE
AND BREAD ON AN ALPINE
MEADOW IN SWITZERLAND

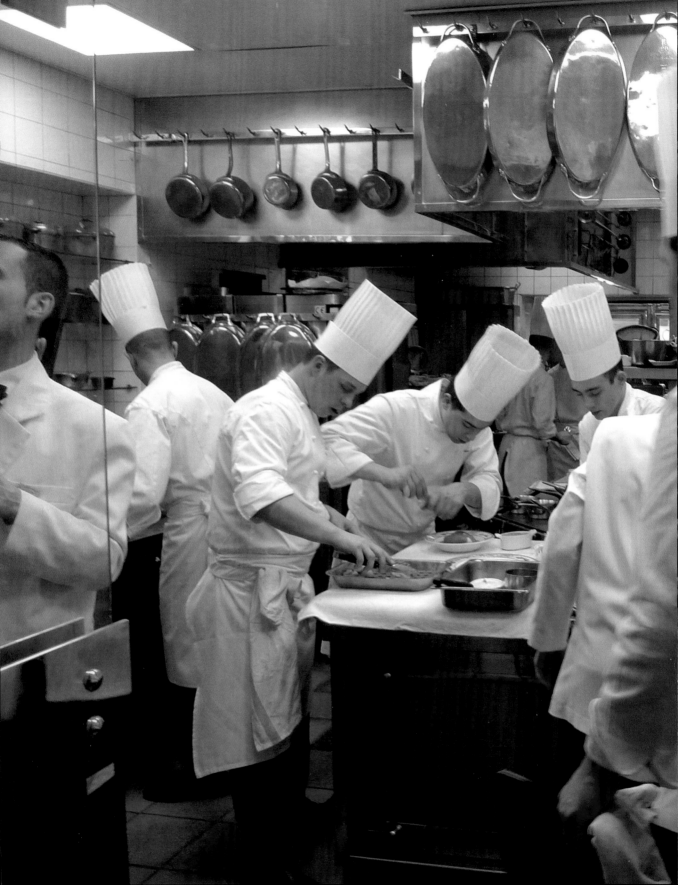

Chapter 5

WHAT TO EXPECT BEYOND THE MEDITERRANEAN DIET

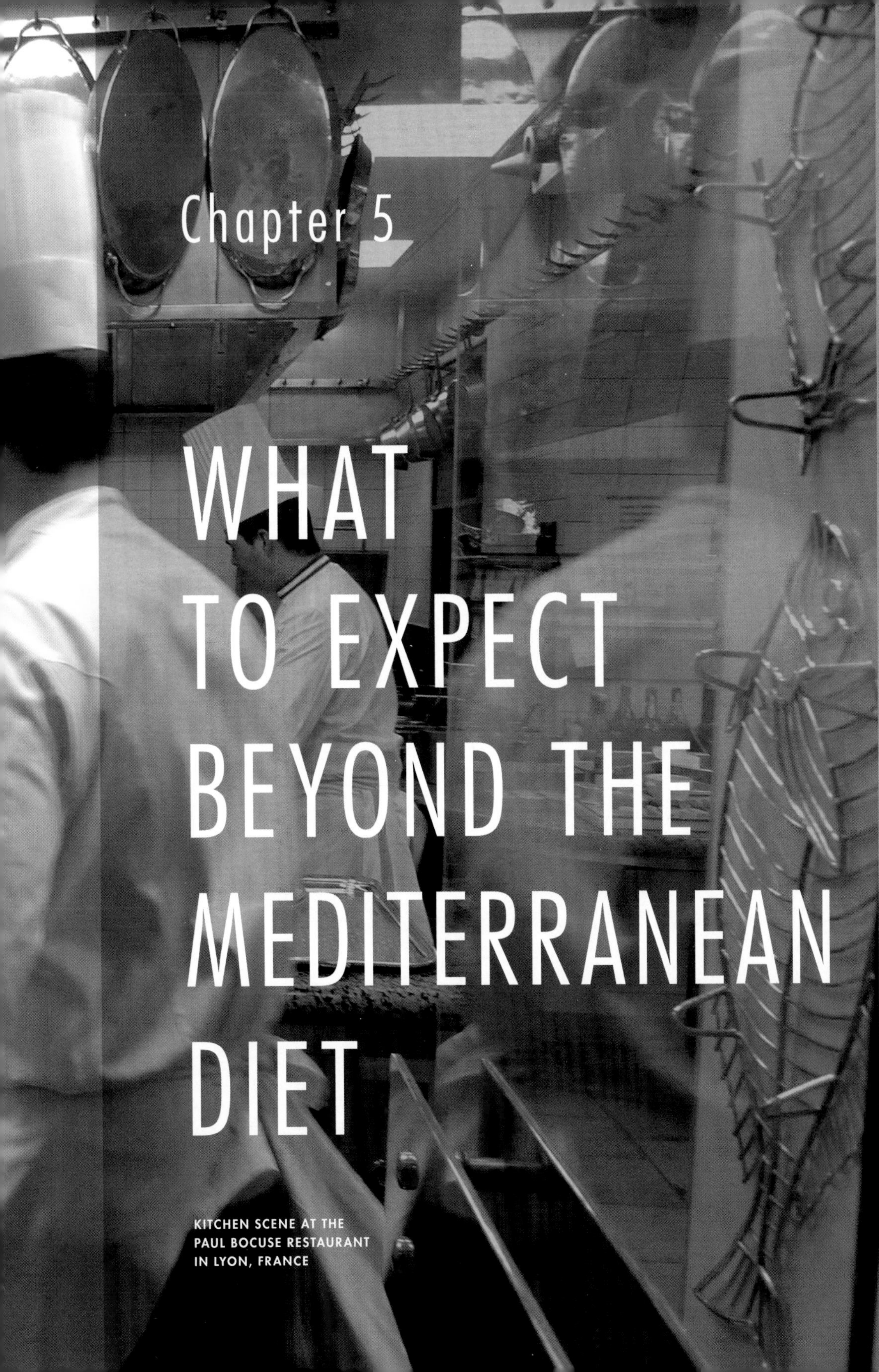

KITCHEN SCENE AT THE
PAUL BOCUSE RESTAURANT
IN LYON, FRANCE

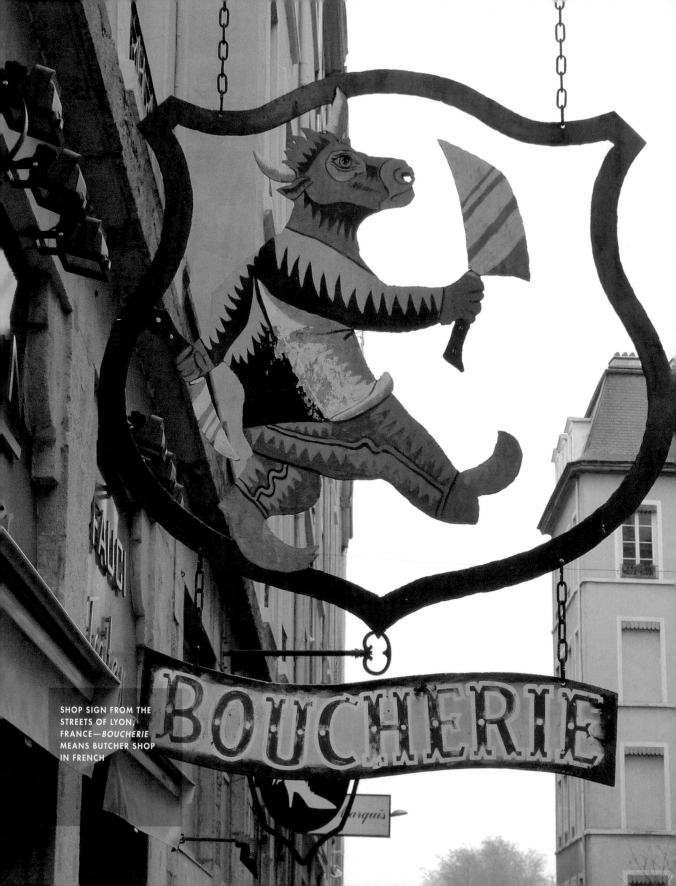

SHOP SIGN FROM THE
STREETS OF LYON,
FRANCE—*BOUCHERIE*
MEANS BUTCHER SHOP
IN FRENCH

The Mediterranean diet, first publicized in 1945, described a specific group of people—the Greeks and southern Italians—who lived in the area around the Mediterranean Sea. It was discovered that these people boasted a longer life span and a lower incidence of heart disease than the norm.

How did they achieve such good results? At the core of their good health was believed to be a diet, coined "the Mediterranean diet," that consisted mainly of grains, vegetables, fruits, beans, nuts, seafood and olive oil. This group ate only moderate amounts of poultry, dairy and red wine, and rarely ate red meat.

For a long time, these people resisted the lure of modern food and drink found in wealthier industrialized countries, such as America, which glorifies the consumption of meat and fast foods. Ironically, as these nations began to choose "convenience" foods, their rates of heart disease, obesity, diabetes and certain cancers rose.

Today, the people of Crete, the largest Greek island, continue to consume large quantities of olive oil, but they have succumbed, unfortunately, to a more westernized way of eating. McDonald's opened there in the early 1990s, so Cretans' current diet mainly consists of meat, processed cheese and sweets, with a heavy dose of television-watching thrown in! Greece now has the second highest rate of childhood obesity in the world—after the U.S.

In America, the influence of food advertisements and our "car culture" with its lack of a physically active lifestyle make it even more difficult for us to follow the diet and habits of the original Mediterranean diet. However, the conveniences and advantages of modern life, when used wisely, can certainly benefit our health and well-being.

For example, thanks to improved transportation and agricultural progress, America has a wider variety of healthy food choices available to almost everyone. Consider today's abundance of fresh fruits, vegetables and low-fat dairy.

Those who lived in the Mediterranean regions during the 1940s, 1950s and 1960s actually depended on what they produced locally. And while the media tried to entice Americans to follow the Mediterranean diet, it was a struggle to maintain it. There are just too many temptations and choices in our modern diet to stick to such a traditional one. Therefore, obesity, heart disease, high blood pressure and diabetes continue to flourish in our country.

Now, *Beyond the Mediterranean Diet* offers readers an easy way to find the right balance between convenience and health, using the best of European dietary habits as a model. It's easy to stick to the principles of *Beyond the Mediterranean Diet,* because you can satisfy your taste buds with a wide variety of foods and get slim and healthy at the same time.

Thanks to the media, the Mediterranean diet was inaccurately described soon after its appearance. Rather than focusing holistically on the need to eat more fresh foods and less meat and packaged foods, the media and advertising simplified the message by focusing on individual components of the diet, such as olive oil instead of butter, with its high levels of saturated fat. Olive oil is known to be heart-healthier, because it contains mostly monounsaturated fat, which may promote heart health.

Soon, the food industry jumped in, and suddenly grocery store shelves were overstocked with a variety of olive oils—including highly processed ones. Because Americans tend to believe "more is better," we not only began to deep-fry foods in olive oil, we even bathed in it! (Yes, there are olive-oil soaps.)

However, Americans missed the fact that olive oil is pure fat, the most concentrated source of calories in our diet. Because of our less active lifestyle and our tendency to eat large portions, it's best for us to reduce all types of fat. Our focus should be on choosing foods that are less calorically dense, including: complex carbohydrates like vegetables, fruits and whole grains; lean protein and low-fat dairy.

Here is what to expect *"Beyond the Mediterranean Diet"*:

1. THE RIGHT AMOUNT OF FAT

America's pursuit of the Mediterranean diet increased the amounts of monounsaturated fat (and total fat) in our diets and lined the pockets of the olive oil industry. Unfortunately, it did not improve our obesity statistics. The Mediterranean diet recommends 35 percent of calories from fat. However, like most American food recommendations, there is no limit on *total calories or calories from fat, just percentages!* Too much of any fat makes you fat!

To obtain the right balance of fats and in the right amounts, *Beyond the Mediterranean Diet* recommends eating plant-based whole foods that naturally contain essential fatty acids. Sources include dry-roasted or raw nuts and seeds, natural nut butter (nothing extra added*), olives and avocados. Cold-pressed oils, like extra-virgin olive oil, are to be used in moderation.

Animal and whole-milk dairy fats like filet mignon, butter and cream should be used in small amounts and less often. (Remember, Julia Child told us, "Don't be afraid of a *bit* of butter!)

Our sedentary American lifestyle and habit of eating larger quantities dictates that total fat intake should not *exceed* 25 percent of calories, which is more than enough for the body to absorb essential fatty acids and feel full. Fat is calorically dense—more

(*For example, reduced-fat peanut butter may contain salt and sugar to boost flavor.)

than twice as many calories as carbohydrates and protein. For example, if you eat 1,200 to 1,500 calories per day, that equals 30 to 40 grams of fat per day.

For example:

• One tablespoon of peanut butter contains 100 calories and eight grams of fat.
• One quarter of an avocado contains 60 calories and six grams of fat.
• One tablespoon of olive oil contains 120 calories and 14 grams of fat.
• Five small, Greek Kalamata olives contain 45 calories and four grams of fat.

Since fat has more calories (nine calories per gram) than other components of food, the 10 percent lower fat in the *Beyond the Mediterranean Diet* can actually prevent obesity. According to dietary guidelines, healthy adults over age 19 require only 20 percent of calories from fat. Most foods contain some quantity of fat. If you eat a well-balanced, whole foods diet, you may not need to add fat to your diet.

Alcohol contains seven calories per gram.
Carbohydrates and protein, each contain four calories per gram.

2. DAIRY AND DAIRY ALTERNATIVES PLAY A ROLE

The Mediterranean diet limits dairy by recommending a moderate intake of eggs, cheese and yogurt. It does not recommend milk or milk alternatives such as almond, oat, soy or rice milks. In the Mediterranean, from 1945 through the 1960s, only full-fat dairy products were available. It was not until 1988 that lower-fat milk products gained widespread acceptance and exceeded whole milk sales.

Today there are many varieties of low-fat dairy products and dairy alternatives, including organic, fat-free, low-fat and reduced-fat milk, yogurts and cheeses. Eating low-fat dairy and enriched, non-dairy alternatives provide protein, calcium, vitamin D and other nutrients, and most importantly, allows us to enjoy these foods. In fact, switching to low-fat dairy is more nutritious than the full-fat version, because it is higher in calcium. Choose organic varieties to avoid added hormones and pesticides.

By limiting dairy, which is suggested by the Mediterranean diet, those who need calcium and vitamin D for strong bones and blood pressure control are being short-changed. Compared to the more active outdoor lifestyle of the Mediterranean people back in the '50s, Americans do less weight-bearing activity to strengthen their bones and have less exposure to sunlight, limiting their ability to produce that valuable vitamin D.

Beyond the Mediterranean Diet recommends three daily servings of low-fat or fat-free milk, yogurt and enriched dairy alternatives. Research confirms that a high intake of low-fat dairy can lower blood pressure, prevent osteoporosis and aid weight loss. Yogurt with live cultures maintains the right balance of bacteria in your intestines. Eggs (egg whites and up to four egg yolks per week) and low-fat cheeses are recommended as part of your daily protein intake.

3. MEAT MATTERS: QUANTITY AND QUALITY

The Mediterranean diet limits meat to just a few times per month. This no longer makes sense, because today's meat is now available leaner than ever before, due to modern breeding programs and new trimming techniques. While most Americans believe that meat is packed with artery-clogging saturated fat, half the fat in beef is actually heart-healthy, monounsaturated fat. In particular, beef contains oleic acid, the same type of fat that's found in olive oil.

Since the 1980s, in the U.S., the pork industry is controlled by a small number of companies that are *not* animal-welfare approved. In the news recently, a company from China purchased the largest pork producer in the U.S. Concern has been raised regarding the impact this will have on U.S. food safety. Therefore, when it comes to pork, buy it pasture-raised and organic from a reputable farm.

Nutritionally, meat contains a wide range of vitamins and minerals, especially iron. Around 20 percent of women and 50 percent of pregnant women lack sufficient iron in their bodies, putting them at risk for anemia. This condition causes extreme fatigue, lack of energy and shortness of breath when exercising. Eating meat is an easy way to obtain iron, even though there are other equally good sources such as oysters, clams, mussels, shrimp, sardines, cooked soybeans, pumpkin seeds, quinoa, blackstrap molasses, tomato paste, white beans, cooked spinach, dried peaches, prunes and lentils.

Beyond the Mediterranean Diet recognizes that the positive attribute of meat does not outweigh the overall negative impact of an American meat-rich diet. However, the problem with meat lies with our excessive portions and low-quality choices. We favor steakhouses that serve a pound or more of fat-marbled steak that was dipped in butter and then char-grilled. A steakhouse's typical 16-ounce beef tenderloin has 58 grams of fat and 912 calories (not including the butter). A popular burger has 630 calories and 35 grams of fat. And did you even count the onion rings? One small serving equals 320 calories and 16 grams of fat!

Do you recall the "pink slime scandal" when an alien-like ingredient coined "pink slime" was uncovered as an additive in the processing plants of ground beef? Pink slime was originally used in pet food as filler and was actually approved for *limited* human consumption.

Buyers beware of ground meat that says lean or 90 percent fat-free, which is based on weight, not the percentage of calories from fat. Four ounces of lean ground beef contains 199 calories and 11 grams of fat. Given that there are 9 calories in each gram of fat that equates to 99 calories from fat, which is about 50 percent fat—doesn't sound lean to me! In most ground chicken and turkey products, all parts are ground up, including skin and bones. Therefore read the ingredients and make sure the label says ground skinless and boneless breast only.

Because of these practices, *Beyond the Mediterranean Diet* urges you to choose your meat (and poultry) carefully. Know your sources and choose local, organic and grass-fed or pasture-raised varieties. Favoring organic meat guarantees that no antibiotics, hormones or genetically engineered organisms are intentionally used. Choose lean cuts and avoid ground meat and poultry unless the butcher grinds it in front of your eyes. It's also best to buy a whole chicken rather than chicken parts. (A whole is less processed than its parts.)

A four-ounce portion of top round steak contains 188 calories and nine grams of fat. A four-ounce portion of pork tenderloin contains 154 calories and six grams of fat. A four-ounce portion of skinless chicken breast contains 120 calories and one-and-a-half grams of fat. Eating smaller portions of high-quality meat and poultry allows you to enjoy meat as part of a well-balanced diet.

In summary, *Beyond the Mediterranean Diet* emphasizes portion control and recommends a daily total of three to four ounces (for women) and five to six ounces (for men) of *extra-lean* animal protein, or a combination of extra-lean animal and vegetarian proteins. (See Appendix for What Counts As One Serving.) Remember it's ideal to choose grass-fed meat and pasture-raised poultry that are also certified organic.

As to portion size, the palm of your hand holds about three ounces. Trim off visible fat before cooking and opt for cooking methods that don't require extra fat to be added, such as steaming, baking, poaching and roasting. Avoid charring meat, which creates cancer-causing compounds.

Now, let's get started with the most important tool so you can begin to go *Beyond the Mediterranean Diet*: "The Super-Healthy Plate!"

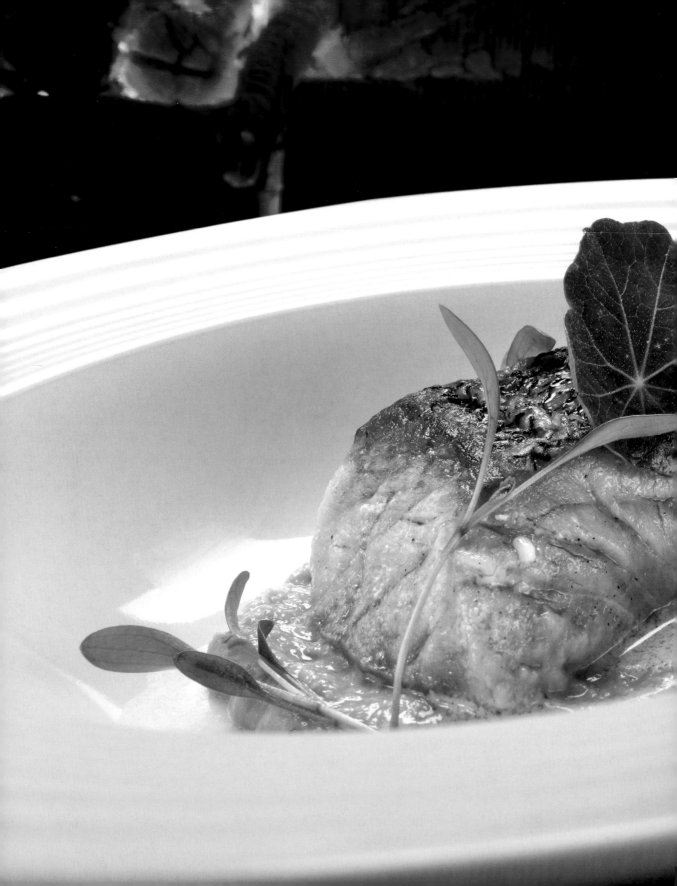

Chapter 6

SIZE *DOES* MATTER—TOSS OUT THOSE LARGE PLATES

HAUTE
CUISINE

ORGANIC   GMO FREE

LOW FAT   FRESH

SUPER-
HEALTHY
PLATE

NATURAL   LOCAL

BIO   VITAMINS/MINERALS

F eel like shopping for some new dishes? Great! I'm giving you permission to ditch your old dinnerware and get some new, healthier-size plates. Not only will you replace those old plates with some brand-new ones, but if you follow my suggestion, you may lose that unwanted weight, too!

Times have changed since our grandparents' day, when a dinner plate was the size of what we now call a "salad plate." Since then, the size of a dinner plate has gone up a whopping 23 percent, from nine inches to 12 inches, and the more food you put on your plate, the more calories you'll consume. While this doesn't seem like much of a difference during the course of one day, if you add up all those extra calories, you could be eating 500 to 1,000 calories more a day. If you consume an extra 500 calories per day, that adds up to 3,500 calories, or one pound of fat, per week. Now imagine that pound of yellow, rubbery fat going from your plate and into your body—every week!

And there's more—since the 1980s, food manufacturers supply us with around 700 more calories per day, thanks to added fat and sugar in packaged foods. If you eat an extra 700 calories per day, seven days a week, that equals 4,900 extra calories. One pound of fat is equal to 3,500 calories. That's over another pound of fat per week!

Many studies have proven that we are influenced by optical illusions when it comes to how much food we eat. This is called the "Delboeuf Illusion," which gives us a false perception of the size of items. A Cornell University researcher found that those who use small dishes serve themselves 12 percent *less* than they intended, and those who use large dishes serve themselves 13 percent *more* than they intended. The good news is, we can use the illusion of more food to our advantage.

Just to satisfy your curiosity, find a ruler or measuring tape and measure the size of your salad plates. Are they close to nine inches? If so, meet your brand new dinner plates! If they're smaller, it's time to replace them with new nine-inch plates, your "Super-Healthy Plate."

Color matters, too. Being able to distinguish color differences on your plate (red, green, white, yellow and orange) will actually make you feel more satisfied when you eat them. The *contrast* between the color of the food and the color of the plate, or the color of the plate and the color of the table, is equally important.

For example, if you are serving pasta with white sauce on a white plate, you are more likely to serve too much food, compared with serving pasta with red sauce on a white plate. Contrast is important to the eye.

When serving chicken and mashed potatoes (white food), pick a colorful plate or a clear glass plate with a colorful placemat underneath to create the contrast.

When serving salmon with black quinoa, use a white plate or a clear glass plate with a white tablecloth so you can clearly see your food. You'll eat less.

107

When you go shopping for those new nine-inch plates, consider clear (see-through) glass plates. That way, you don't have to change your plates, just your placemat or tablecloth color. Make sense?

While you're busy measuring your plates, get out your drinking glasses, too. It's so easy to indulge in too much of a sugary drink, such as fruit juice. The best serving size for juice is a four-ounce glass, so take out your glasses and fill up your liquid measuring cup. Then, see how this amount looks in your juice glass. If it looks tiny, your glasses are too big. If it looks just right, then your eyes and your tummy will adjust to that portion size. (To save calories, pour only one ounce of juice in the glass, and fill the remainder with sparkling water.)

Here's a tip: When you're ready to buy new drinking glasses, choose tall, skinny ones. This is an optical trick called the "T-illusion." We tend to overestimate the length of a vertical line relative to a horizontal line of the same size. According to Cornell University researcher Brian Wansink, even professional bartenders pour more in a wide glass and underfill a tall glass.

Better yet, follow the European approach to enjoying juice and squeeze two medium size oranges into a small juice glass. This will produce about four ounces of fresh orange juice, exactly the right amount. Four ounces of juice contain 56 calories and 11 grams of sugar, compared to 112 calories and 22 grams in an eight-ounce glass. Keep in mind that four grams of sugar equal one teaspoon, so four ounces of juice equal almost three teaspoons or one tablespoon of sugar!

In 2009, the American Heart Association recommended no more than 100 calories or about two tablespoons or six teaspoons (25 grams) of added sugar per day for women and 150 calories or about three tablespoons or nine teaspoons (38 grams) for men. Overall, it's better to get sugar from eating whole fruits, because its natural fruit sugar is gradually absorbed, thanks to the fiber. Otherwise, the sugar in fruit juice alone produces a rapid rise in blood sugar.

In addition, you'll receive more nutrients and trace minerals when you eat whole fruits compared to just the juices.

The size of a "standard" portion on the label of a family-size juice or milk carton will always say eight fluid ounces. However, for single-serving bottles, cans and cartons, the portion is one serving, and the container size dictates that portion. So a 20-fluid-ounce bottle of Coca-Cola is one serving at a whopping 260 calories and 65 grams of sugar. A 14-fluid-ounce, single-serve carton of Tropicana orange juice is considered one serving at 190 calories and 39 grams of sugar.

This reflects a food-labeling law back in 1997 that standardized serving sizes of packaged foods. No doubt this has helped widen our waistlines, and it may explain why we drink far more juice and soda than Europeans do.

Beverage labels in Europe limit portions to 100 milliliters (ml), or 3.38 fluid ounces. Going from a European portion of 3.38 fluid ounces to an American portion of 20 fluid ounces makes a big difference. It's a whopping six times the amount of calories and sugar!

After the birth of her child, my friend Jane decided she needed to lose 20 extra pounds she'd put on during pregnancy. When she started reading food labels, she realized that drinking a 16-ounce bottle of soda in the afternoon was adding excess calories (200 calories and 55 grams of sugar) but offered no nutritional value. She wanted real food for those calories instead of a high-fructose sweetened drink, so she decided to drink water and eat fresh fruit instead. With this simple change, she felt more satisfied, and no longer had an afternoon energy lull. She's also fitting into clothes she hadn't worn for years!

Next, it's time to give up those oversized dinner forks and tablespoons, and opt for salad forks and teaspoons. Try three-pronged appetizer forks for dessert and teaspoons for soup. When you eat with a smaller fork or spoon, it's harder to gobble down your food. Therefore, you'll linger over your meal long enough for your brain to register that your stomach is actually "full" about 20 minutes after eating.

How is this advice European? Europeans use smaller dishes and utensils than we do, and they don't eat supersized portions. Therefore, a French sandwich with two to three ounces of meat or cheese on a nine-inch plate would look pretty small on one of our 12-inch plates. Your eyes and stomach would complain: Is *that* all I'm getting? I need more than *that*!!

THE SUPER-HEALTHY PLATE

The "Super-Healthy Plate" is a simply designed, yet powerful portion-control guide to encourage Americans to create healthier, more relaxed mealtimes. Your new nine-inch plate can be used for any meal or snack—and it's far easier to lay out the appropriate helpings of healthy, delicious food that you'll be preparing in Part Three.

By using the nine-inch plate, you can control portions without having to weigh and measure food. Clearly this is preferable to having to carry around a food scale! It's also a fun way to create your own menus, using the plate as a guide.

Wine should be consumed European style: in moderation, sipped slowly with meals. You can substitute various forms of alcohol, such as exchanging four ounces

1.

WATER

SKINNY CAPPUCCINO

TOMATO

WHOLE-GRAIN SOURDOUGH

PART-SKIM RICOTTA CHEESE • JAM

FRESH ORANGE

REDUCED SCALE
EXAMPLES OF SUPER-
HEALTHY PLATES FOR:

1. BREAKFAST (PAGE 172)
2. LUNCH (PAGE 186)
3. SNACKS (PAGE 200)
4. DINNER (PAGE 214)
5. DESSERTS (PAGE 228)

2.

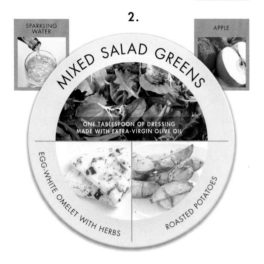

SPARKLING WATER

APPLE

MIXED SALAD GREENS

ONE TABLESPOON OF DRESSING
MADE WITH EXTRA-VIRGIN OLIVE OIL

EGG-WHITE OMELET WITH HERBS

ROASTED POTATOES

3.

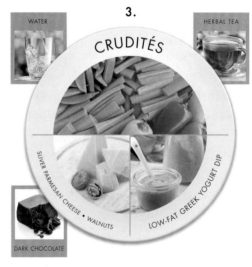

WATER

HERBAL TEA

CRUDITÉS

SILVER PARMESAN CHEESE • WALNUTS

LOW-FAT GREEK YOGURT DIP

DARK CHOCOLATE

4.

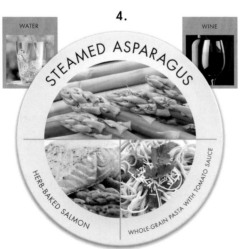

WATER

WINE

STEAMED ASPARAGUS

HERB-BAKED SALMON

WHOLE-GRAIN PASTA WITH TOMATO SAUCE

5.

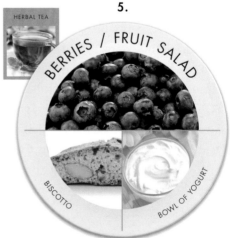

HERBAL TEA

BERRIES / FRUIT SALAD

BISCOTTO

BOWL OF YOGURT

of wine for one ounce of vodka or eight ounces of "lite" beer. By the way, beer bottles in Europe are typically 11.2 ounces, not the 12 ounces common in America! Alcohol content of different beers, wines and distilled spirits can vary, so read the label. (See Appendix for more information about alcohol.)

If you are trying to lose weight, limit yourself to 16 ounces of wine (or equivalent) per week! Heavy drinking can lead to increased risk of health problems such as liver disease, gout, elevated triglycerides, brain damage and breast cancer. Women are more sensitive to the effects of alcohol, because they have lower body fat, fewer enzymes to break down alcohol and hormonal changes. Furthermore, if you have medical conditions or take medications, consult with your physician and pharmacist to determine if alcohol is off limits.

Like alcohol, sugary sweets and greasy fats are empty calories and should be carefully portion controlled.

The "Super-Healthy Plate" will help you start eating like a European. This design encourages you to eat more vegetables and get the right proportions of other foods.

As you can see, the plate is divided down the middle. One half is dedicated to a variety of your favorite non-starchy vegetables and salads. The other half is equally divided between proteins and starchy foods. For snacks, yogurt often replaces protein or starch. For dessert, fruit replaces vegetables.

Side dishes that surround the breakfast, lunch and dinner plates are fruits, beverages, low-fat yogurt/milk, plus occasional indulgences like a square of dark chocolate or a four-ounce glass of wine.

Proteins include fish, extra-lean meat, poultry, cheese, dry-roasted nuts, beans, lentils, tofu, eggs, etc.

Milk includes low-fat milk and yogurt and alternatives like enriched almond, rice or soy milk/yogurt.

Starchy foods include potatoes, pasta, rice, couscous, quinoa, corn, green peas, lima beans, grains, bread, cereals, etc.

Non-starchy vegetables include carrots, broccoli, cabbage, green beans, cauliflower, spinach, Swiss chard, turnips, beets, etc.

Fruits include berries, melon, fruit juice, applesauce, pears, kiwis, apples, figs, dried fruits, canned fruits, etc.

The reason non-starchy vegetables are given half the plate's "real estate" is because—whether raw, roasted, steamed, microwaved or baked without added fats—they are the least caloric, most nutrient-dense foods, providing fullness and quantity with fewest calories. Adding more non-starchy vegetables into a recipe or cooking with tomato- or vegetable-based sauces will have the same impact. The Harvard School of Public Health recommends five to 13 half-cup servings of vegetables per day. The "Super-Healthy Plate" guide will get you there!

Let's start with breakfast, with tomatoes taking up half the plate as the non-starchy vegetable. Whole-grain sourdough bread (starch) takes up one quarter of the plate, and part-skim ricotta cheese (protein) takes up the other quarter. If you prefer a sweeter breakfast, add a tablespoon of fruit jam for the bread.

Around the plate, there is a sliced orange (fruit) and a skinny cappuccino (coffee made with steamed low-fat milk). Notice the orange is sliced. This encourages slower eating and longer enjoyment of the fruit.

Remember, if you have an eight-ounce glass of water with your meal, it will help your stomach feel full faster. This breakfast plate sends a clear message: Drink water and eat fresh fruit, rather than drinking from cartons of pasteurized juice.

For lunch, a mixed green salad is the non-starchy vegetable component and takes up half the plate. Roasted potato (starch) is one quarter, and a three-egg-white omelet (protein) is the other quarter. Around the plate are an apple and, always, a glass of water—flat or sparkling. For children or if you want to increase calcium, consider a smoothie: blend one cup of milk with one cup of fresh fruit. That's all that's needed for a satisfying, naturally sweet, delicious and nutritious shake! (You can add ice if you like it cold.)

For the snack, *crudité* (assorted raw or slightly steamed, cut-up veggies) takes up half the plate as the non-starchy vegetable. Here, we forgo the starch in favor of a sliver of Parmesan cheese or a one-inch square of reduced-fat cheese and three to four walnuts (protein). These occupy one quarter of the plate, and low-fat yogurt dip (dairy) fills the other quarter. Around the plate you see herbal tea, water and, if you must, a small piece of dark chocolate.

This snack is aimed at someone who is trying to lose weight. For kids or those who feel like they need more food, add a serving of starch, such as three graham cracker squares, a half sandwich or one of the snack recipes in Part Three.

For dinner, asparagus takes up half of the plate as the non-starchy vegetable. A three- to six-ounce filet of grilled salmon (protein) is one quarter, and one cup of whole grain pasta (starch) with tomato sauce (more veggies) takes up the other quarter. If you wish, add a four-ounce glass of red or white wine, and always add a glass of sparkling or flat water. As a general guide, if you're trying to lose weight, the average man should consume no more than six ounces of cooked salmon, while the average woman should consume half as much, or three to four ounces.

Two to three hours after dinner, if you're craving dessert, enjoy fruit and yogurt or a biscotto with herbal tea. Alternatively, see recipes in Chapter 14 for a sampling of healthy, yet decadent desserts.

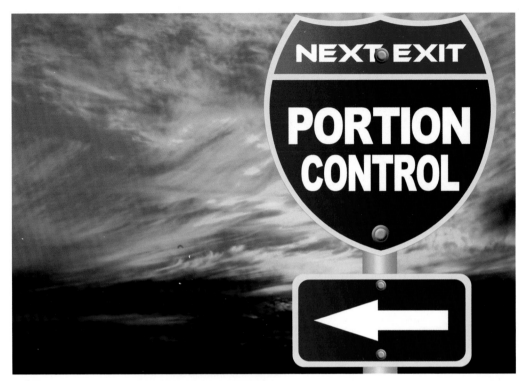

EMBRACE PORTION CONTROL AS A LIFESTYLE

The nine-inch plates shown here are *guides* to help you make healthy food choices while avoiding oversized portions. Use your best judgment when making substitutions and when foods are mixed together. When available, choose fresh, local, organic, natural and sustainable ingredients. Season your food with herbs and spices, rather than salt. (See Appendix for Herb and Spice Seasoning Guide.) Use fresh fruit, dried fruit and fruit sauces instead of sugar. If you must use a fat, choose cold-pressed, extra-virgin olive oil, even with bread. Use butter in small quantities only when it's worthwhile, such as tangy, nutty French butter from Normandy or a local artisan brand.

When eating meat, choose lean cuts and remove the skin from poultry. At least half your starchy foods should be whole grains, such as brown rice or starchy vegetables like peas or potatoes—not potato chips, which are processed.

Dairy should be low-fat or fat-free. You can use alternatives such as enriched soy-milk, almond milk, oat milk or rice milk.

For those on special diets or with specific nutrient needs, like pregnant and lactating women, please consult a registered dietitian and physician before making dietary changes. Keep in mind that portion size varies depending upon your caloric needs, weight, height and activity level, so use your best judgment.

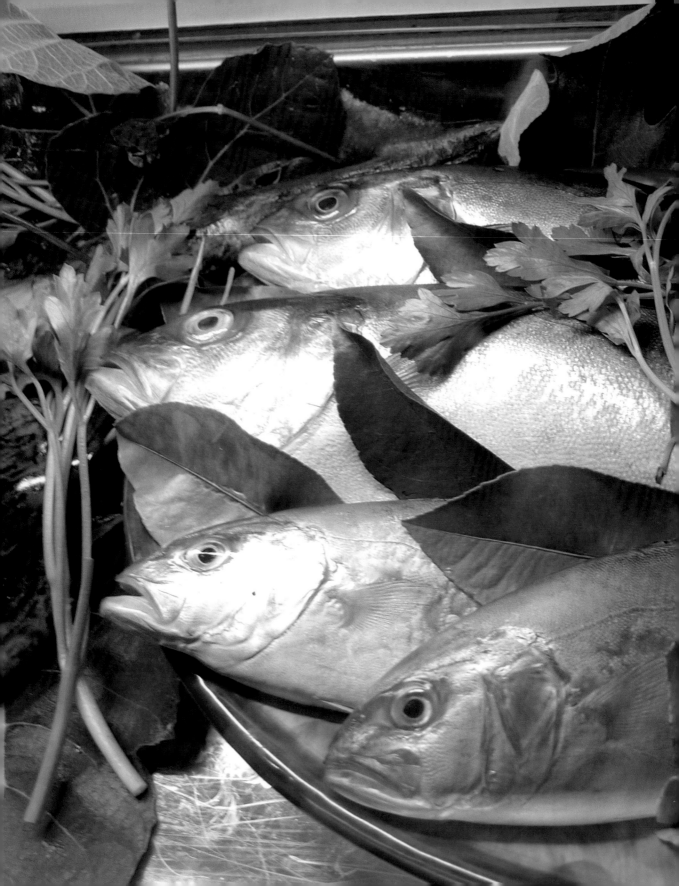

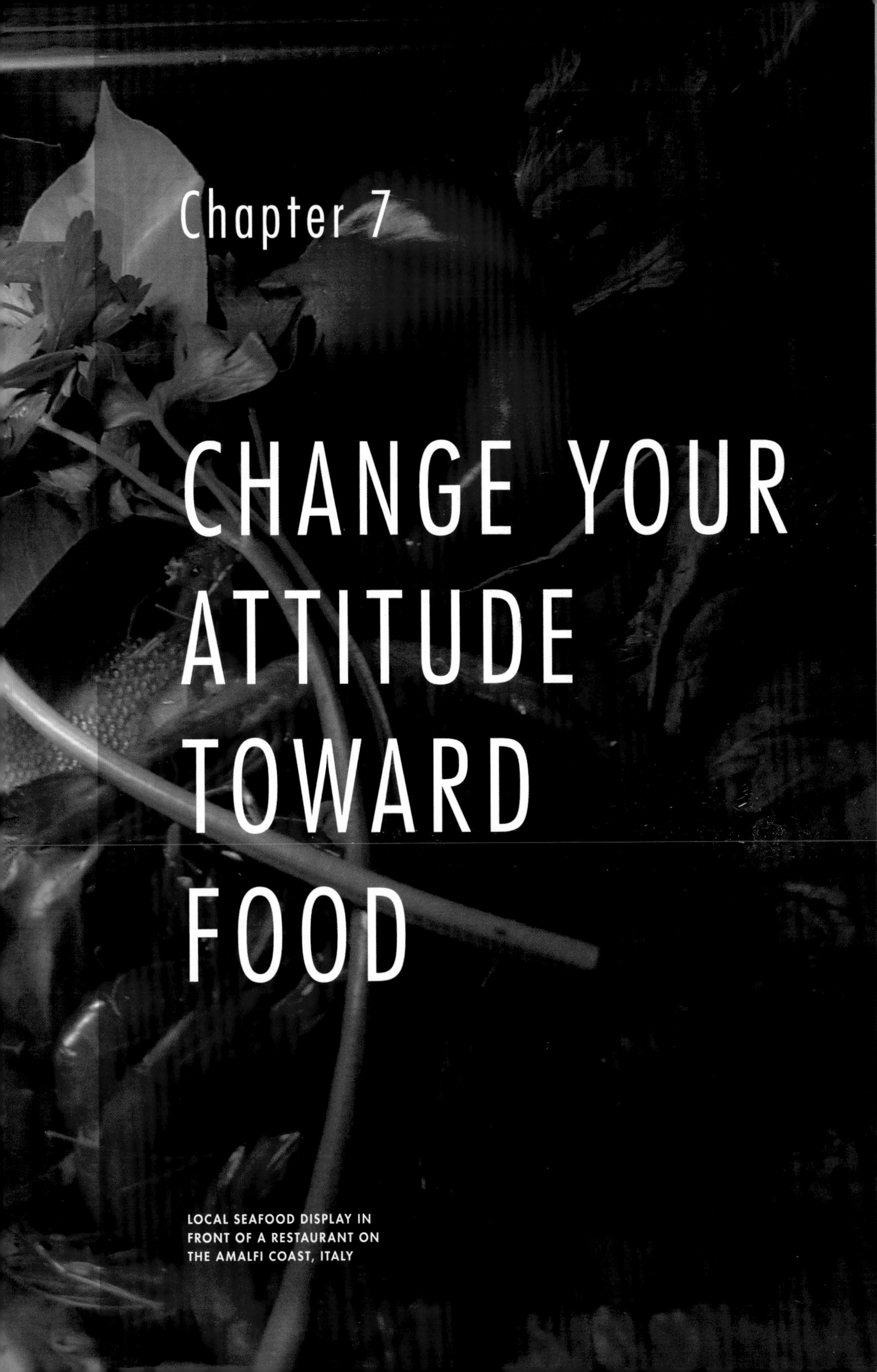

Chapter 7

CHANGE YOUR ATTITUDE TOWARD FOOD

LOCAL SEAFOOD DISPLAY IN
FRONT OF A RESTAURANT ON
THE AMALFI COAST, ITALY

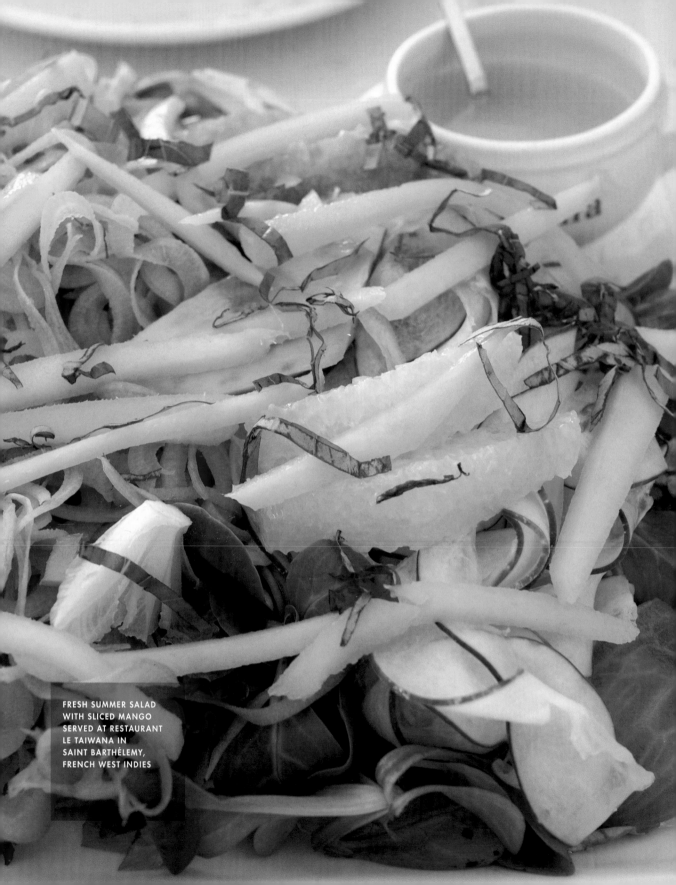

FRESH SUMMER SALAD
WITH SLICED MANGO
SERVED AT RESTAURANT
LE TAIWANA IN
SAINT BARTHÉLEMY,
FRENCH WEST INDIES

The key to success in shrinking your belly is to develop new dietary habits and behaviors that make you feel 100 percent in charge of what you eat. Since you're the person who chooses "what and how much," you need not rely on a server or a food manufacturer, or fall into the trap of the chemists, scientists and marketers who are working to get you hooked on specific kinds of food.

Our "grab and go" culture offers us another trap. Everywhere you look, you're encouraged to "hurry up and eat." This is the opposite of Europe's attitude of "relax and linger." In fact, back in the 1980s, an Italian named Carlo Petrini began "The Slow Food Movement" to prevent fast foods from infringing on his country's beloved food culture. Today, the movement is firmly entrenched in Europe and spreading worldwide. Now, Italians, Swiss and French would never dream of gulping down a meal. They chuckle at the "Big Gulp" ads and wonder how anyone can enjoy that "green thing" that causes you to burp every hour.

Rushing through your meal means that your stomach has not had enough time to signal to your brain that it's actually full, since it takes at least 20 minutes for your brain to register that your stomach is full. To slow down your intake, use smaller utensils, take mini bites, chew more and linger between each taste. Time yourself. How long is it taking you to eat a plate of food? Does it normally take you only five minutes? Set a timer for 20 minutes, so you know when to expect your brain to register fullness. Now, relax and enjoy your meal—just like a European!

There are other ways to take the edge off your hunger. Start your meal with a non-creamy vegetable or broth-based soup or a large green salad (with dressing on the side). These appetizers will fill you up a bit and help curb your appetite. Consider enjoying an herbal tea with your meal. (In European countries, it's called an *infusion*.) Because a hot drink requires small sips, you'll be forced to slow down. If you sip a relaxing herbal tea like chamomile midday or in the evening, you'll find you're more relaxed and less tempted to binge in the afternoon or evening.

STEP 1: REJECT THE LURE OF LARGE PORTIONS

Restaurants follow the trends of the multi-national fast food chains that are training Americans what and how they should eat. Independent restaurants then feel pressure to serve large portions too. The problem is that if a large plate of food is set in front of you, it's a cue to eat more of it. Distractions or "multi-tasking" also contribute to overeating. Examples include watching TV, a movie or texting, which often results in a lack of focus on the enjoyment of the food. Eating often becomes "mindless" and uncontrolled.

117

Today, almost every supermarket has a "Grab & Go" case filled with prepared foods, to compete with fast food chains and convenience stores. For example, when you are commuting home from work, you may want a little something to tide you over until dinner. That's when "Grab & Go" might come in handy, if you make a thoughtful choice.

A European might choose a small sandwich with one-ounce of cheese and one-ounce of meat amounting to 175 calories. In comparison, an American may grab a hero sandwich with two ounces of cheese and three ounces of meat amounting to 425 calories. A European portion is smaller and in line with what's actually needed. So order a half sandwich, or take half home. You'll get used to it once you try it. Besides, who would want to feel overstuffed *before* dinner?

OUT OF SIGHT, OUT OF MIND: IF YOU SEE IT, YOU'LL EAT IT!

Tempted to dip into some of your favorite goodies in the pantry? Out of sight, out of mind works! First, identify what your weaknesses are, then remove them from your house. My colleague, Dan, can't even think about turning down ice cream, so he simply doesn't keep it in his freezer anymore.

If you can't control how much chocolate you eat when it's in the house, give yourself a once-a-month treat and stick to one small piece. On a positive note, keep that healthy food, such as a tempting bowl of fruit, at eye level on the kitchen table. If you see it, you'll eat it!

STEP 2: TRAIN YOUR PALATE

Those small bumps you see on your tongue when you say "ahhh" hold the secrets to your taste experience. They are called *fungiform papillae*. Buried within them are your taste buds. Taste buds also exist in other places like the throat, mouth and stomach. They allow you to distinguish sweet, sour, salty, bitter and savory tastes.

The average person has between 2,000 and 10,000 taste buds, and those with more than 10,000 are called "supertasters." Supertasters tend to dislike sweet desserts and bitter vegetables, finding them too sweet or too bitter.

While taste buds are responsible for distinguishing just a few tastes, flavor—a combination of taste and smell—detects hundreds. The sense of smell is responsible for 75 percent of what we call "taste." There is also a difference between smelling through your nostrils (inhaling) and smelling using your mouth (exhaling). So both the taste buds on your tongue and the passageway in your nose are essential for becoming a connoisseur of great-tasting food!

The more you can sharpen your taste buds, the more you'll turn into a super taster. In fact, you'll cringe at the thought of wasting valuable calories on high-fat, high-sugar, overprocessed, nutritionally worthless food! Let's look at how you can enhance your ability to taste, get the most flavors, and savor each bite.

The practice of eating simply prepared food will help you more easily identify specific ingredients. Your sense of taste is stronger when your brain receives images of food through your eyes. Have you ever looked at a window of pastries and felt pleasure without even touching them?

Did you know that the sense of smell is improved after you exercise? Even a brisk 10-minute walk counts! It is likely linked to an increase in nasal moisture after a workout. And if you live in a dry environment, in order to keep your eyes and nose lubricated, consider a humidifier, especially in winter. A moist nasal passage will sweep up the aroma of good food long enough for your brain to say, "Thank you. I am satisfied!"

It makes sense that drinking water throughout the day, even hourly, is not only important for satiety and hydration, but also for your ability to taste. Having a dry mouth will impede your taste buds. Just like your nose, your mouth needs moisture to maximize taste, so stay hydrated, six to eight cups a day keeps the appetite at bay!

Make sure you're getting enough zinc, because a lack of this mineral in your diet is linked to loss of taste. The amount needed varies depending upon age, ranging from two milligrams to 12 milligrams per day. Too much is not good either and can cause low copper, low immunity and low HDL cholesterol.

Oysters are an excellent source of zinc and contain 74 milligrams per three-ounce serving. Other good sources include three ounces of beef, crab or lobster, ½ cup of baked beans and ¾ cup of fortified breakfast cereals. The amount of zinc in these foods varies from three to seven milligrams per serving. Eat foods that contain zinc. Besides, eating food is more enjoyable than popping a pill!

Hundreds of medications are known to affect taste and smell including statins, antidepressants and high blood pressure medications. It's important to talk to your pharmacist about your regimen and ask about side effects including weight gain, water retention and increased appetite. There may be alternatives to your medications, so the conversation is worthwhile. By following this diet, chances are you'll soon be off the meds anyway.

Managing colds and allergies is essential to keeping your palate in good working order. If you catch a cold, gently blow your nose and try to keep it unblocked. Good food is like a breath of fresh air only when you can breathe easily and smell the roses! If allergies are an issue, see an allergist who can prescribe the proper medications to help you breathe and taste better. Inhale and exhale deeply, and you will suddenly feel fulfilled!

Smoking damages the nerves in the back of your nose, so give it up! And stay away from second-hand smoke and prolonged exposure to stinky smells like dirty diapers, which will ultimately lessen your sense of smell.

Very hot foods and liquids can damage your taste buds. That's why it's better to eat most foods at room temperature. For example, the volatile oils of cheeses are released at room temperature, not at cold temperatures. The same is true of red wine. Granted, coffee's aroma is better hot, but not burning hot!

Always eat when you're hungry, because that's when your sense of taste works the best! You may want to try adding spices to your food like chili powder or red pepper flakes. Spices stimulate the nerve that makes you cry when you cut an onion. Using spices will get you off fat and salt while enhancing flavors.

Keep an eye on the quantity of wine and alcohol you consume at a meal. The ability to smell lessens as blood alcohol rises. Plus, too much alcohol leads to mindless eating, dehydration and excess calories!

We know that thoroughly chewing your food will prolong the meal, giving your brain more time to register fullness. More chewing also allows food to linger in your mouth. The longer you linger, the more foods will mingle with your taste buds. Before you put a forkful of food into your mouth, stir it on your plate to release the aromas so your nose can identify the smells. It's a good habit to smell everything you eat and drink. This will improve your sense of smell overtime.

A technique that's proven to improve taste, is to take a bite of a different food with every forkful, rather than mixing it all together or eating one food completely before going onto the next one. This keeps the olfactory nerves from getting bored and keeps the taste experience more exciting.

If your current diet is high in fat, sugar and salt, you probably can no longer detect them, because you're so used to them. I have a favorite trick to get you off fat, sugar and salt. It has worked for everyone who has tried it. Choose one food you eat regularly with a high-salt content. For example, if your cereal has 200 milligrams or more of salt per serving, switch to a brand with less than 50 milligrams per serving. Do this for at least two weeks. Now switch back, and you will be stunned by the taste of the high-sodium cereal. This also works with sugary and fatty foods.

STEP 3: BECOME A FOOD SNOB

Europeans are said to be snobbish about food, but in truth, they appreciate and take pride in high quality food. This does not equate, by the way, to choosing and preparing more expensive food.

For example, the price of potato chips is almost twice the price of carrots or potatoes for the same portion. A pot of herbal tea is less expensive than an equal quantity of soda. And being able to eat the skin of an organic apple in comparison to having to peel the skin off a conventional apple makes the organic apple more cost effective. In addition, the skin actually offers more nutrition and fiber.

Bake your own low-fat chips: In a roasting pan, toss two to three cups of thinly sliced carrots and potatoes with one to two teaspoons of extra-virgin olive oil. Cook at 400 degrees Fahrenheit for about 35 minutes.

Fine food and quality ingredients are for everyone, even for children. School lunch menus in France, Italy and Switzerland are made with the same ingredients that patrons pay good money for in fine restaurants. European kids dine on the same food as their parents, like steamed mussels, roasted potatoes and stuffed artichokes. These children grow up to be adults with healthy eating habits.

In the U.S., kids' menus featured in schools and restaurants are highly processed (high in fat, sugar and salt), featuring fried chicken nuggets, hot dogs and tater tots. The food industry has us believing that our kids won't eat other types of food; nothing could be further from the truth! In fact, children who are exposed to wholesome, healthy foods, like fresh fruits and vegetables, actually prefer these over fast foods.

Being a "picky eater" or a "food snob" doesn't have to do with being negative about certain foods. It's actually about being selective about which foods you prefer to eat. You deserve to have it all—nutrition, freshness, wholesomeness and satisfaction!

Instead of an Egg McMuffin, make your own scrambled egg whites with roasted pepper and feta cheese, served on a whole-grain English muffin. This can easily be done in the microwave in less than three minutes. Check out the healthy egg recipes in Part Three.

Think of the word "pairing" to create good, creative dishes. For example, if you want to eat more fresh fruits, think about how you can add them to other foods to be creative. For example, microwave a banana for two minutes and serve it over yogurt with a dash of cocoa powder. Or serve a sliced apple with a square of low-fat cheddar cheese. If you need more veggies in your diet, consider dicing mushrooms and peppers into tomato sauce. Or serve salmon over steamed baby kale.

Insist on fresh ingredients so that complex preparations aren't needed. Start sampling seasonal foods. Try new versions and enhance old favorites, using herbs and spices rather than sugar and salt. For example, if you love strawberries, dice and toss them with a splash of balsamic vinegar instead of sugar. When strawberries are out of season, consider using frozen varieties and add them to smoothies. Frozen fruits and vegetables are typically frozen during peak harvest, so they are good alternatives when fresh are out of season.

The food regulatory agencies make it easy for food producers to sell consumers all sorts of things that may not be good for us. Therefore, we owe it to our families and ourselves to become educated consumers. With knowledge and awareness, we have the ability to make better decisions that will help protect our family's health.

Enjoy being a leader as a locavore—someone who eats locally produced food. In addition to favoring local food, consider also being an organic steward. All organic food is non-GMO (non-genetically modified organisms or crops) and rBGH-free. Conventional dairy often has rBGH hormone added, unless it says otherwise on the label. It's best to lower your exposure to added hormone so as not to upset your own body's natural production.

Supporting producers who take pride in delivering high-quality, unadulterated food that tastes great naturally is rewarding. Just bite into a strawberry that was grown close to your town, lovingly nourished in organic soil, and picked the day before. It'll taste so much better—and provide more vitamin C—than a strawberry that was flown or trucked in from a long distance, covered with pesticides and preservatives!

STEP 4: EAT WHEN YOU ARE HUNGRY

I'm sure you've heard the term "calories in equal calories out." It is the total number of calories you consume that will ultimately determine if you lose, gain or maintain weight.

The problem is, we often eat too many calories, because we haven't developed a pattern that satisfies our hunger. Instead, we become used to eating even when we are *not* hungry. Then we eat again when we *are* hungry! Some of us don't even know what hunger feels like!

The first thing you can do to reverse this trend is to keep a food diary. Try it for at least three days, and preferably a week. Write down everything you eat and drink, including the time and accurate amounts. Jot down notes about how you are feeling— hungry, tired, bored? Also include the times you exercise, and what kinds of lifestyle activities you engage in, such as walking or gardening. Once you identify your patterns and habits, you can modify them. For example, if you eat chips at 10 p.m. because you are watching the news on TV, replace them with a pot of herbal tea to help you sleep. Keep in mind that physical activity does *not* give you the right to then "pig-out."

With practice and attention to your unique hunger signals, you will learn what time, how much, and types of foods you should be eating. Weekends may be easier to try this, so gather the family and work out a plan for meals together. It's important to strategize about when to eat and how much food you'll need. For example, if you have special dinner plans, be sure to lighten up at lunch with a soup or salad and a half sandwich.

My girlfriend, Amy, is a mother of two young girls who come home from school famished. Within an hour of arriving home, the girls consume an enormous quantity of healthy food (fruits, vegetables, whole grains, cheese and/or yogurt). At dinnertime, they eat a modest portion, unlike their mother, who is starving and grabbing seconds, because she didn't have an afternoon snack. Amy has consulted with me, and we both agree that it's wise if she joins her daughters with a mid-afternoon snack, so she isn't overeating at dinner. Thus, she can use more calories during the day, rather than at night when her body wants to slow down.

Consider a snack a mini-meal, and include the same high-quality ingredients you would eat at a regular meal. For example, eat half your sandwich at lunch with a salad. Eat the other half in the late afternoon with fresh fruit.

123

Talk show hosts tell you to fast one day and eat anything you crave the following day. In other words, starve and binge. Shouldn't you be listening to what your body is telling you, rather than listening to a TV host? Starving and binging can upset your body's metabolism, resulting in inefficiency in burning calories. This leads to weight gain and the yo-yo dieting syndrome. One day on and one day off, always trying a different fad, can result in weight fluctuations, but doesn't produce steady weight loss.

Don't skip breakfast. This lowers your blood sugar and will make you jittery and unable to concentrate, and can also create the urge to binge later on. You'll find it difficult to make healthy food choices when you're starving, and you'll be tempted to cave into cravings. Breakfast should be a light meal of cereal, fruit and milk, or a slice of toast with fresh cheese and tomato to help you "break-the-fast." Check out Chapter 10 for some deliciously simple breakfast recipes.

STEP 5: TURN OFF THE TV, COMPUTER AND CELL PHONE, AND INVITE A NEIGHBOR FOR DINNER!

Unlike our Italian friends who love to socialize over the dinner table, we spend too much time eating alone, rushing our meals, and missing out on the taste of our food. "Grab, Gobble and Gulp" is hardly the recipe for enjoying our food!

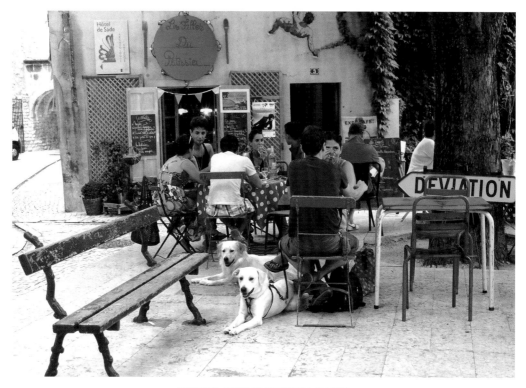

OUTDOOR SCENE IN PROVENCE, FRANCE

124

By sharing mealtimes and savoring food with friends and family, we feel far more satisfied on many levels. Research shows that those who socialize more are less likely to become obese. Europeans set a fine example of focusing on healthy food, good company and a comfortable mealtime setting.

Many Americans eat on the run or choose to eat from a tray, lost in a favorite TV show and barely tasting the food itself. Here's some advice: If you want to become slender and healthy, turn off the TV, computer and cell phone at mealtimes! In fact, make sure to leave all electronics far away from the dinner table. Eating is supposed to be a shared activity to create memories of love, laughter and companionship. One way to achieve this is to invite family and friends over. Research has confirmed that eating with someone else can actually make your food taste better!

Be sociable when eating with others. Conversation helps slow down the meal; that means your brain can tell your belly when it's had enough. If you are eating alone, treat it as sacred time and make your place at the table as attractive as when you entertain guests. Digestion works better in a pleasant, relaxed setting.

For example, my friend, Lisa, received a thoughtful card game gift called "Table Topics." Those around the table would pick out a card and discuss what was on it: from your favorite childhood movie to your most embarrassing moment. Such conversations can create great memories of pleasant mealtimes.

If you're single, make plans with neighbors and friends, or join a dining club. Today, many restaurants, cafes and markets have a "social" or "community" table filled with people you don't know. When you're out with other people, you're more likely to be on your best behavior and not go for that third helping of pie! Usually, when we're in public, we show more restraint and better etiquette.

Believe it or not, it's also a good idea to eat with men! College students of both genders who eat in the presence of men actually eat less, according to researchers.

Preparing a meal can be enjoyable, too. Turn on your favorite relaxing music, light candles and have the kids set the table. If you don't make enough time to share your daily rituals, you'll lose the opportunity to practice what's important as a family. These activities also create your own "Slow Food movement" at home, which encourages your family to be more conscious of how and what they eat.

It's time to regard meals as more than a time to consume food: It's also a time for love, laughter, companionship and fun!

125

STEP 6: YOU DON'T NEED A GYM TO GET MOVING!

It's time to get physical! Europeans love lifestyle activities—and their trim bodies confirm it. The French recommend "moving around" for at least 30 minutes each day. The Swiss agree, and favor outdoor activities to indoor ones. Both Swiss and French are fond of Pilates, a method developed over 70 years ago to increase flexibility and core strength. The Italians are a bit less gung-ho when it comes to activities, but they love sports and are soccer fanatics.

Europeans are not gym enthusiasts, however, and gyms and fitness centers are quite unpopular throughout Europe (with the exception of Pilates centers).

In general, Europeans include lifestyle activities into their daily lives. Those who live in small cities and villages walk or bicycle to most places. Driving to restaurants, shops and parks is less common in Europe, where you can walk to so many places.

We Americans are, alas, at a disadvantage when our own government guidelines recommend that adults have a minimum of two hours and 30 minutes of "moderate" aerobic activity per week, or one hour and 15 minutes of "vigorous" aerobic activity per week. Nowhere do the guidelines define "moderate" or "vigorous." Nor is there any mention of sports or lifestyle activities like bicycling, walking, gardening or swimming, which can also burn calories.

Upon further research, I found out that the CDC does define "moderate" and "vigorous" activities. Moderate activity includes: walking at a brisk pace of three to four-and-a-half miles per hour on a level surface or outside like walking the dog or bicycling five to nine miles per hour outside or indoors on a stationary bicycle. Other activities include yoga, calisthenics, weight training, dancing, swimming, kayaking, horseback riding, gardening, shoveling light snow and moderate housework.

Vigorous activity includes: race walking at five mph (miles per hour) or faster, jogging, hiking on an incline, mountain climbing, bicycling more than 10 mph or on a steep hill, high-impact aerobics, jumping jacks, boxing, singles tennis, competitive sports, whitewater rafting, shoveling heavy snow and heavy housework.

Ultimately, it all comes down to one simple fact: whichever form of exercise you choose, you'll lose one whole pound after you've burned 3,500 calories. That's about 10 hours' worth of moderate intensity exercise. Moving around more, useful as it is, will not do the trick unless you eat less, too. And rewarding yourself with beer and chips after a vigorous workout is not a good idea.

Having a scheduled activity plan is the first step. First, see your doctor to obtain medical clearance. Commit to at least 30 minutes every day—even if it's a 10-minute walk three times a day, it counts. Learn about the importance of cardiovascular (running, cycling, walking), strength (weight lifting, resistance training, Pilates) and flexibility (yoga, stretching) training, so you can participate in all types of activities.

You may want to hire a personal trainer to set up a program, but you don't need a gym to do it. Physical activities can be done in your home using a treadmill, exercise ball or a stationary bicycle. You may also choose to go to yoga or Pilates classes. A simple walk in the park or at a mall can be planned at least a few times a week.

Like Europeans, try to include other lifestyle activities throughout the day. Instead of driving, walk to do an errand or park the car a mile away. Toss a ball on the beach, play an instrument, make your bed, clean the house, pull some weeds, wash your car, push a shopping cart and cook dinner.

Share your strategies with a "weight-loss buddy." This can be a friend you confide in, who will hold you accountable for sticking to your new approach. Schedule daily walks together and document your activities and food intake in a diary.

Beauty sleep will help you eat better and improve your level of physical activity and endurance. People who are sleep-deprived eat more fat and sugar to stay alert. When you're tired, your brain cannot focus to make good decisions, so the better you sleep, the better you eat.

Aim for eight hours a night. You can get there by being physically active during the day. It's more effective than sleeping pills to ensure a good night's rest. That trio of sleep, exercise and eating well are essential in ensuring a long, healthy life.

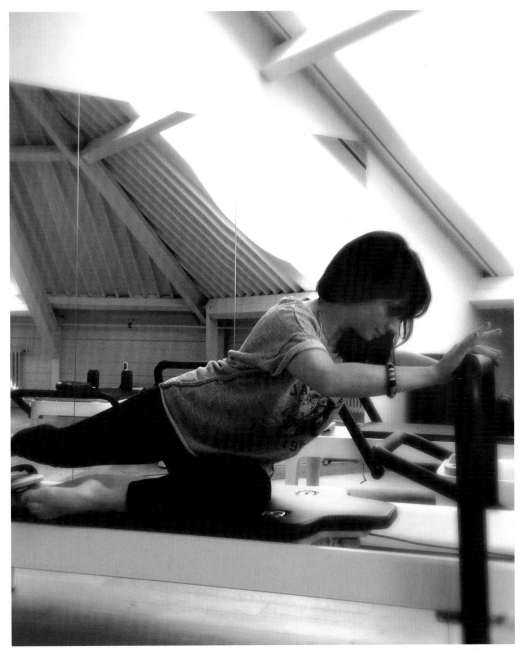

OLIVIA PLISSON, MY FRENCH PILATES INSTRUCTOR AT MOVEMENT FACTORY IN CAROUGE, SWITZERLAND

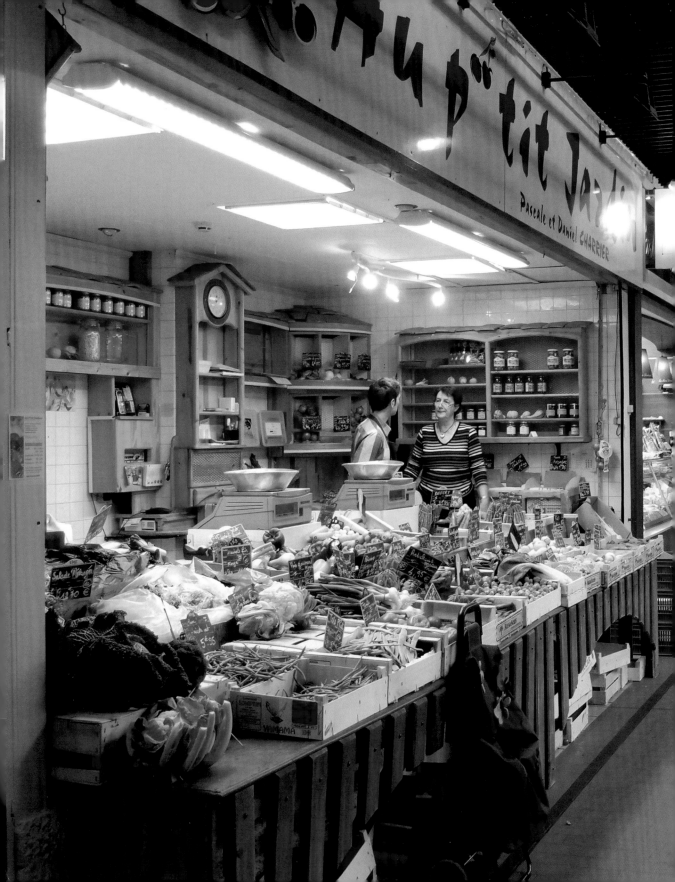

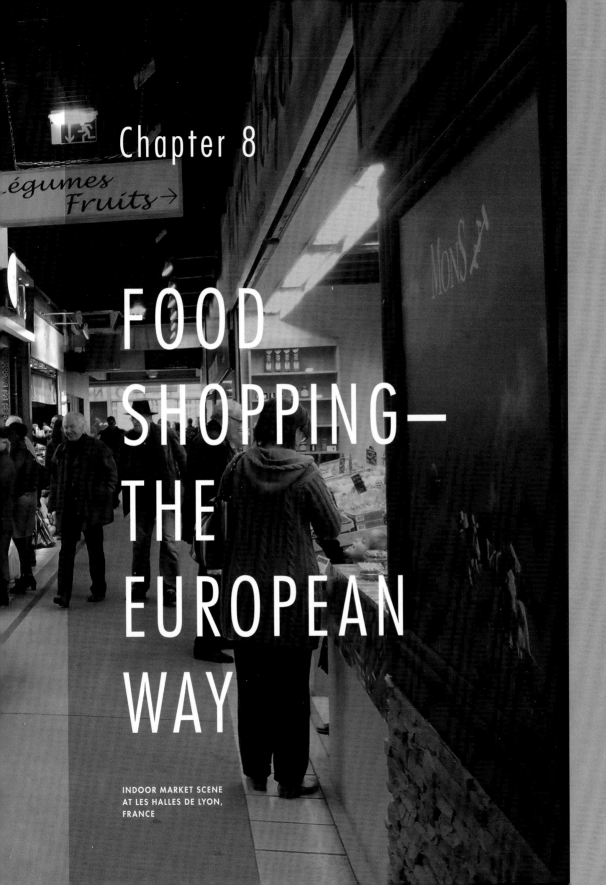

Chapter 8

FOOD SHOPPING— THE EUROPEAN WAY

INDOOR MARKET SCENE
AT LES HALLES DE LYON,
FRANCE

buy
local

FRESH PRODUCE AT A
LOCAL FARMERS MARKET

There's no doubt about it. Compared to Europeans, we Americans must be alert when we go food shopping. Otherwise, we find ourselves seduced into buying food that may do us more harm than good. In order to dodge the maze of potentially dangerous foods laced with GMOs, pesticides, additives, chemicals and preservatives, reach for natural, organic, local and unprocessed food. That makes it easier to avoid falling prey to the food industry's game of hooking us into buying deceptively advertised unhealthy food.

Europeans don't have to contend with this problem, because their supermarket shelves are stocked with more natural and less processed foods. The latest energy drink or trendy cupcake or cookie offering does not easily impress them.

Even though our food labels tout more health claims than you'll find on European food labels, there are ingredients lurking inside those packages that you would not want to consume. That "low-fat, low-sugar" pound cake *might* sound healthy, but it likely contains white flour and artificial sweeteners. Health claims make us believe that it's good for us. But ask yourself: "Do I really want to pay for empty calories and laboratory produced ingredients?"

Because our food industry is more of a free-for-all, and marketers are crafty, it's easy to believe bogus advertisements using misleading and meaningless words like *skinny, sports, vitamin* and *power*. Many brands of these so-called "healthy snacks and beverages" including enhanced water, energy bars and gluten-free bakery products are often no better than sugary drinks, candy bars and conventional snacks.

Lately, every TV show host and Hollywood celebrity is telling us what to buy, what to eat and what to cook for dinner. While apparently well meaning, these people are not registered dietitians and may be getting paid for endorsements. So take their advice with a "grain of salt."

Let's take a look at how you can best ensure that what you choose is not detrimental to your health and is, instead, safe, nutritious and delicious.

MERGE FRESHNESS WITH CONVENIENCE

There are several differences between shopping European style and shopping American style.

First, geography plays a role. European cities and villages have existed for centuries, and farms were always nearby to serve the community. Because transportation was not as modern as it is today, people ate locally. There was a local butcher for your meats and a baker for your breads and sweets. It was easy to run out and get a fresh loaf of bread from the corner baker, or stop by the butcher to pick up a roast for dinner.

Every Saturday, a farmers market would come to town, where one could buy fresh fruits and vegetables in season.

Second, Europe is more densely populated than America. Because of a lack of space for housing, European dwellings are smaller and have less room for huge appliances and food storage. Because markets with fresh foods are available nearby, there is no need for large refrigerators and huge amounts of food to be stored at home.

America was developed much differently. Because we have a greater land area, there is a greater distance between cities and towns. With the arrival of cars, the suburbs sprang up, often far from the existing markets and bakers. Even today, people often drive long distances to get to a market to stock up on food.

In the U.S., local farms were often sold to accommodate the increased demand for housing, giving rise to small pockets of commercialized farm industries throughout the country, the biggest one being in the state of California. The food industry convinced us that big-box stores were more convenient and economical than "mom and pop" operations—a very different scenario in Europe.

Today, Europeans go to supermarkets for staple items like dried beans, grains, oils, dried herbs, flour, sugar, paper goods, cleaning supplies and to bring in fresh food during the week. European supermarkets have a good working relationship with their local farmers, and stock fresh meats and produce because that's what their patrons expect.

Compared to the U.S., European supermarkets carry more fresh foods, fewer "junk" foods, and more organic choices. They make it a point to sell local and organic products at fair prices. Organic foods in America cost twice as much as conventionally produced food, but that's not so in Europe.

While Europeans have access to more fresh foods, we Americans have access to more "convenience" and packaged foods. Convenience is what we thrive on, but it's to our benefit to choose convenient foods that are fresh and natural, like yogurt, pre-cut veggies, apples, bananas and baby carrots. For more elaborate foods like soups, sandwiches and salads, try the "Grab & Go" section in natural food markets.

Take the time to explore and get to know your neighborhood stores and markets that sell fresh food. Make it a point to visit them as needed, and don't overstock. Remember, quality food tastes best when it's fresh—and has more nutritional value!

SHOP MORE OFTEN

Consider the size of European refrigerator and freezers. Compared to our American versions, they're *tiny*. In city dwellings, they often fit under a countertop and measure not more than 10 cubic feet. In the U.S., they'd be considered dorm-size, rather than family size! Compare this to the average American refrigerator measuring 18 to 26 cubic feet.

When I lived in Europe, I got used to the "small fridge phenomenon" and became a regular shopper of fresh food, sometimes daily. While the thought of a daily trip to a food market sounds a bit excessive, daily food shopping ensures that vegetables and fruits don't get old and lose their nutritional value. It also helps us cut down on that bad habit of throwing food away when it's been sitting around too long.

REMEMBER, YOU GET WHAT YOU PAY FOR!

We Americans are always looking for a good deal. Coupon clipping has become a national obsession, with "extreme couponers" strategizing to drastically reduce the size of their grocery bills. However, most coupon offers are unhealthy processed foods: sodas, cereals, cookies, crackers and chips. Have you noticed that organic vegetables, fruits and meats are rarely on sale in conventional supermarkets?

Europeans—whether wealthy or low-income—expect to pay more money for good quality food. They aren't looking for cheap or discounted food. Instead, they realize that quality food is best for their families and that the benefits outweigh the small increase in costs.

133

During high school, my youngest son Alex lived in Spain on a study abroad program and stayed with a Spanish host family. The family lived on a moderate income, yet it was important that every day they enjoyed fabulous, healthy meals together. They looked forward to going to the market for the largest shrimp they could find as a centerpiece in their homemade *paella*. They often planned weekends to include a trip to the country for quality cured ham called *Jamon Iberico*. Before living in Europe, my son had never eaten cured meat or pork. While there, he tried everything and learned to appreciate the local foods.

Have you ever eaten a croissant made by a baker who can create an exceptional one? It's a tedious process to make a croissant, and the recipe calls for a lot more butter than you'd be comfortable eating. When you buy one from a good bakery in France, the flaky pastry, crispy on the outside and doughy soft on the inside, melts in your mouth.

Now, compare that peak experience with a croissant from your local American supermarket. It looks delicious, even though it's packaged in the bakery aisle, so you know it hasn't been baked from scratch in the store.

Still, you're craving a croissant. The color is right, it looks flaky and buttery, and it is a good value. Four croissants for four dollars—perfect! But when you bite into this mass-produced croissant, you're deeply disappointed. It does not taste fresh: It tastes like cardboard with chemicals. Four-hundred (or more) calories later, you've had an unhealthy, unsatisfactory eating experience.

Wouldn't you have preferred a delicious, freshly baked croissant instead of one that was just tolerable? No doubt the rest of the packet of croissants will be tossed out at the end of the week, even though they still look remarkably un-aged. The point is, you would be satisfied just to have a few bites of one delicious croissant anyway!

Americans are used to quantity at a cheaper price, like a BOGO (buy one, get one free) promotion. However, when you seek quantity, you often forfeit quality. The same phenomenon occurs when you seek convenience, because it costs more to produce a convenience food.

The "bargain" involves more packaging, less food and, often, lower-quality ingredients. For example, have you ever looked at the ingredients on a box of flavored rice? I dare you to pronounce or decipher the list. In addition, a two-ounce serving has a whopping 840 milligrams of sodium.

For about the same price you can buy a six-ounce box of plain brown rice with only 10 milligrams of sodium. You are paying for those high-sodium flavorings that were produced in a lab. Besides, using your own fresh herbs and seasonings results in a fresher and more delicious taste.

Convenience and processed foods are costly, and you don't get quality for your money. Instead, you pay for packaging, additives and marketing. In addition, mass-produced foods often lack freshness, because they are pumped up with shelf life stabilizers and preservatives.

The secret to getting the most for your money lies in buying wholesome, organic ingredients in bulk, which are less expensive than their canned counterparts. A one-pound box of dried, organic beans costs $3.68 and makes about seven cups of cooked beans. That's about 50 cents per cup. A 15-ounce can (about two cups) of organic beans averages $2.99. That's about $1.50 per cup, three times more!

If you just don't have time to soak beans, using frozen or canned varieties are indeed convenient. Don't forget to read the ingredients and rinse well to get rid of the salt.

PREPARE A SHOPPING LIST

Europeans shop almost daily for food, but that habit doesn't typically fit into an American lifestyle. Therefore, you must be organized and plan what you "need" before going to the grocery store. Armed with your shopping list, you should be in-and-out quickly with little time for being tempted to buy things you don't need.

Before you go to the grocery store, decide on what you plan to eat for the week. Then, write a list and stick to it. It's fine to be flexible when choosing what's fresh and in-season; just don't be fooled by the tricks of the industry. For example, cross-merchandising whipped cream near the strawberries is intended to tempt you to buy whipped cream when you only planned to buy strawberries. And if you have an impulse to buy that box of cookies piled high at the entry, buy the ingredients instead and make a healthier version at home. Always check expiration dates on perishable foods. To save money on staples, consider choosing generic or house brands.

READ YOUR LABELS: INGREDIENTS COUNT MOST

Read it before you eat it! In the U.S., the nutrition information on a label is called a Nutrition Facts Panel, but in Europe it's just called Nutrition Information. Health claims like "low-fat" or" low-calorie" on packaged foods are unpopular in Europe because Europeans are more concerned about quality ingredients. This follows the European trend of being selective about the food they eat.

It is mandatory, both in Europe and the U.S., for almost all food labels to have nutrition information and a list of ingredients. In the U.S., most of us focus on one or two numbers on the Nutrition Facts Panel and skip reading the ingredient list. However, only looking at the numbers, whether calories, fat, sodium, sugar or fiber, is a big mistake.

Maybe your doctor told you to eat more fiber, so you only check the grams of fiber on a package of bread. Did you ever think that fiber could be coming from added wood pulp instead of from a whole grain? That's why it's important to read the ingredient list.

The list of ingredients is the best indicator of how healthy and wholesome a food is. If what you are buying contains more than five ingredients, or a lot of unfamiliar, unpronounceable items, consider leaving it behind.

Ingredients are listed in descending order of their amount in the food. If fat, salt, sugar and/or refined flour are one of the first three ingredients, chances are the product is unhealthy. (Obviously, this rule doesn't apply when you are buying prepared foods made with wholesome ingredients that are naturally high in fat, such as nuts, seeds and avocados.)

Be sure to check packaged foods for sodium content. (Table salt is sodium chloride.) Too much sodium can lead to high blood pressure. The daily recommendation for sodium is no more than 2,300 milligrams per day, which is 2.3 grams. For those who are older or who already have hypertension, sodium intake should be limited to 1,500 milligrams, or 1.5 grams per day.

135

It's wise to aim for a 1:1 ratio of calories to sodium. For example, if a product has 170 calories per serving, the sodium should be around 170 milligrams. Salt is also a hidden component of other ingredients, including monosodium glutamate, natural flavors, soy sauce, Worcestershire sauce, sodium benzoate, sodium phosphate and hydrolyzed vegetable protein.

We already know that Americans consume too much sugar, which is easy to do if you eat packaged foods. Many fat-free or low-sodium foods will actually contain more sugar. For example, fat-free cakes tend to be composed of mostly white flour and sugar.

Sugar goes by many names on an ingredient label, including sucrose, fructose, dextrose, maltose, corn syrup, high fructose corn syrup, cane sugar, evaporated cane juice and sugar alcohols like xylitol and maltitol. Avoid all artificial sweeteners (aspartame, acesulfame K, sucralose, saccharin); you're better off with a small amount of natural sugar than anything artificial.

The least processed sugars include organic evaporated cane juice, pure maple syrup, raw honey, organic cane sugar, organic stevia, organic agave, organic blackstrap molasses, organic barley malt syrup, organic coconut sugar and organic brown rice syrup. Unfortunately, food companies are now processing even these natural sugars, so read the ingredient labels and ask questions like where is it from and how is it produced.

According to MayoClinic.com, giving raw honey to infants may cause infant botulism, a rare but serious gastrointestinal sickness caused by exposure to bacterial spores. Infant botulism can be life-threatening.

The general rule is to eat only natural foods and small amounts of sugar. As mentioned earlier, the American Heart Association recommends just six added teaspoons of sugar per day for women and nine for men. There are 4.2 grams of sugar in a teaspoon, so six teaspoons equals about 25 grams of sugar.

A good rule of thumb when buying a cold cereal is to check the Nutrition Facts Panel and choose a cereal with five grams of sugar or less per serving. The first ingredient on a cereal label should be a whole grain like oat bran or brown rice flour.

Sugar is hard to cut down on, so eat like a European and go for quality over quantity. Try having one square of good quality dark chocolate, rather than one king-sized candy bar. Your waistline will reflect your change in size, and your taste buds will be more satisfied too!

FAT: THE NUMBER ONE OBESITY CULPRIT

For overall health, our bodies require the right balance of saturated and unsaturated fats. Unsaturated fats include polyunsaturated (omega-3 and omega-6) and monounsaturated fatty acids. Eating too much fat makes us fat, because fat is the most caloric component of food—more than twice the calories of carbohydrates or proteins.

Fats differ in their level of saturation. *Saturated fats* have been known to raise blood cholesterol. Foods high in saturated fats include butter, whole milk, cream, cheese, meat, poultry skin, lard, palm and coconut oils.

Trans fats are "man-made" saturated fats and are the major contributors to an unhealthy heart. Sources include hydrogenated and partially hydrogenated vegetable oils including shortenings and margarines. Margarine *is* hydrogenated oil. Don't be fooled by all the advertisements that margarine is healthier than butter. It's not! Trans fats are often lurking in commercial crackers, cookies, pies, muffins, pastries, microwave popcorn and fried foods. Avoid it when you can.

Saturated and trans fats are solid at room temperature.
Unsaturated fats are liquid at room temperature.
Solid fats clog up your arteries!

Omega-9 fatty acids (monounsaturated fats) are known to be good for the heart. Sources include olive oil, canola oil, macademia nut oil, avocados and many dry-roasted nuts and seeds.

Omega-6 fatty acids (polyunsaturated fats) are known to be unstable when heated and susceptible to oxidative rancidity if stored improperly. Sources include corn oil, safflower oil and soybean oil. Corn and soybean oil are abundant in processed foods and may be responsible for creating an unbalanced intake of essential fatty acids. It's best to store these oils in the fridge and use them sparingly.

Omega-3 fatty acids (polyunsaturated fats) are known to decrease inflammation in the body and reduce the risk of heart disease, cancer and arthritis. Sources include flaxseeds, walnuts, oily fish and fish oils.

It's important to point out that all cooking and salad oils are a mixture of monounsaturated, polyunsaturated and saturated fatty acids. The predominant fatty acid will determine how it is categorized. (See Appendix for Comparison of Dietary Fats.) Many oils are overprocessed and genetically modified, so buy organic oils that are cold-pressed or extra-virgin olive oil.

It's ideal to consume fat from whole food sources that supply a good balance of essential fatty acids and trace minerals. Examples of whole food fats are nuts that are either dry-roasted or raw, seeds like sesame and flax, and avocados.

Still, fat is not the best source of energy for our bodies. Instead, complex carbohydrates like fruits, vegetables and whole grains provide the ideal bodily fuel.

Total daily fat intake should range between 20 to 25 percent of total calories consumed. (The American Heart Association recommends a more generous range: between 25 to 35 percent.) If you eat 1,800 calories a day, then 25 percent would equate to 450 calories from fat or 50 grams of fat. There are nine calories per gram of fat. Fats are in almost all foods, except for most fruits.

BAN ADDITIVES, PRESERVATIVES, CHEMICALS AND DYES

The U.S. food industry is not as "clean" as Europe's. We have more additives, preservatives and dyes added to our foods. Because we expect foods to have a long shelf life, preservatives are not *only* in our food, but are also in the packaging like BHT (butylated hydroxytoluene) and BHA (butylated hydroxyanisole).

U.S. food companies pride themselves on consistency in taste. In order to maintain consistency, natural and artificial flavors are often added to packaged foods. Even natural food products like cereals and energy bars often contain lab-produced natural flavorings.

Synthetic dyes are derived from petroleum and are cheap, stable and brighter than most natural dyes made from, for example, paprika, beet juice or turmeric. The trend to switch to natural is stronger in Europe, but some U.S. companies like The Hain Celestial Group recognize its importance. Blue Dye #1, popular in sports drinks is banned in France and Switzerland and may cause cancer including brain tumors. Citrus Red Dye #2 used to color the skins of Florida oranges is toxic to animals even in modest amounts.

Potassium bromate, an additive used to increase volume in white flour and breads is banned in the UK, parts of Europe and California, because it causes cancer in animals. Sodium benzoate and potassium benzoate, mold inhibitors commonly found in diet soda, hummus, fruit juice and pickles are known to cause allergic reactions in certain individuals.

*Phosphoric acid in colas erodes tooth enamel, depletes calcium
and is linked to kidney stones.*

The European Union does not allow cows to be injected with rBGH (genetically engineered Bovine Growth Hormone), chickens to be washed in chlorine or arsenic in its chicken feed. Yet, in the U.S., chemical baths of antimicrobial sprays are used on poultry and meat processing lines—as a fix to the problems of E. coli, salmonella and other antibiotic-resistant pathogens! Even organic meat and chicken are often bathed in peracetic acid—an organic compound, which is basically vinegar and hydrogen peroxide. Don't believe that *all-natural* is the essential term to look for on meat, poultry or packaged food labels, because neither the U.S. Food and Drug Administration, the U.S. Department of Agriculture nor the Federal Trade Commission have a strict definition for all-natural.

The list goes on and on, so for more information, see the Appendix for Chemical Additives and visit the website: *http://www.cspinet.org/nah/05_08/chem_cuisine.pdf*

Read your ingredient labels and don't buy anything with an ingredient you don't know. Don't assume that supermarket deli-counter salads or prepared meats are made with natural ingredients. Do your research and get to know your markets, farmers and producers to find out exactly how food is being brought from the farm to your table!

PATRONIZE MARKETS WITH FRESH, ORGANIC AND LOCAL FOODS

With more frequent deliveries and people shopping more often, the food is always fresh in European food markets. Fresh food means better nutrition and optimum taste! Bread is baked daily from scratch and never sold a day old. The wide variety of fresh food sold is chosen for taste and nutrition unlike in the U.S., where varieties of fruits and vegetables sold in supermarkets are based on how well they hold up to mechanical harvesting and shipping.

Think of the transportation costs of fresh strawberries grown in California that are headed to the East Coast going over 2,000 miles, compared with a truck of fresh strawberries coming in from 200 miles or less to villages and cities in Europe. Hauling refridgerated food across the country is not only environmentally unfriendly but results in a lower quality product with fewer nutrients and less flavor.

Europeans choose food according to seasonal availability, so when food is out of season, they either won't have it or will import it from closer places such as Morocco— imported, but still not that far away.

Americans are used to having "seasonal produce" imported year-round. It's often less expensive, because the costs of labor and farming are lower in other countries—even though long-term environmental costs are greater. The reality is that even in winter, it makes more sense to grow cool weather crops like lettuce in a greenhouse rather than pay the high fuel costs of shipping. While we may continue to haul in citrus and bananas from tropical climates, it is irresponsible to buy food that is produced so far away from home.

Have you read the recent news that many of our imported spices have a high risk of salmonella contamination? This is due to poor sanitation and unregulated food processing in non-western countries—giving us more reason to care about where our food is coming from.

Europeans patronize local and artisanal food shops. How could they not? Everything is made from scratch and tastes delicious. They enjoy relationships with the proprietors and know where the meat from the butcher comes from, because the butcher has a long record of satisfaction in the community.

In the U.S., "mom and pop" food shops find it difficult to compete with big-box stores. Even if they want to produce better-quality products made from scratch, consumers refuse to pay the extra costs. For example, bakeries today rarely bake their own breads and pastries. Instead, they bring them in from large factories that mass-produce them. They often finish baking semi-prepared goods and let the aromas waft into the store, giving the impression they are made from scratch. It's an illusion, and you get what you pay for!

When we lived in Geneva, we looked forward to Saturday mornings at the farmers market on Rue de Rive. Throughout Europe, squares are set aside for local farmers to drive their produce into town, as well as for the artisanal cheesemakers, bakers, jam and condiment makers and other small merchants. A wonderful variety of wines, cheeses, fresh breads, seasonal fruits and vegetables were always available.

My husband would especially look forward to seeing his favorite organic wine producer, who only had so many bottles to sell every week. If you weren't there early enough to get one, try again the next time. The grower knows what he or she can comfortably produce in the time that he wants to work. Whereas in America, when an item is advertised and out of stock, we expect a "rain check" on the price of that advertised good. If it's not there when advertised, we know we'll still get it at that price. Not so in Europe.

Buying locally produced food supports local families, preserves open space, benefits the environment and

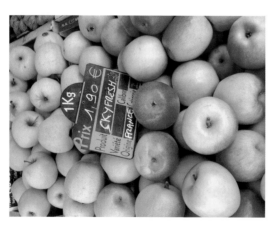

APPLES OF FRENCH ORIGIN

creates a connection to the community. For example, buy your bread from a local artisanal bakery. You may not be able to get there every day like in a European city or village, so buy two loaves of fresh bread—one for now and one for later. Fresh breads and many other items freeze well.

Wrap the bread well before freezing so it retains its moisture. When you're ready for the second loaf, allow it to thaw completely before unwrapping. Then put it in the oven for five to ten minutes at 350 degrees Fahrenheit and enjoy it that day!

In the European Union, it is mandatory for most products to be labeled with "country of origin" including wine, poultry, beef, fruit and vegetables. For example, the sign above the apple display is marked "from Switzerland" or "from France," while the sign above the dates is marked "from Turkey."

In America, the "country-of-origin labels" only recently took effect. Now stores are required to post where meat, poultry, seafood and agricultural products are from, unless they are considered "processed." In this case, processed can mean mixing two or more types of ingredients together like a chicken salad of chicken, celery and mayonnaise. I recently purchased a frozen organic Oregon berry mix from Costco that was recalled for a nationwide hepatitis outbreak. It was discovered that an ingredient in the mix—pomegranate seeds imported from Turkey—were contaminated. Since this was a "mixed" product, and the amount of pomegranate seeds did not meet the quantity threshold for mandatory labeling, the origin was not disclosed on the label. Even I was tricked into believing the berries were from Oregon.

Now that these laws are in place, use them to make informed decisions. Choosing food that is locally and regionally grown helps small-scale ranchers and farmers make a living from the land and helps sustain rural communities.

When I'm food shopping in Colorado and crave fish, I choose freshwater striped bass; it's farmed locally and ecologically. Colorado is known as a meat-producing state, so it's important to know which ranchers are using sustainable and healthy methods of raising cattle. I look for certification from third-party certifiers not linked to the cattle industry. For example, third-party certifiers include Certified Humane, USDA Organic, and Fair Trade Certified. Don't be fooled by stamps of approval by food companies who create their own stamps or buy stamps from industry-backed councils and organizations.

I encourage you to look for farmers markets wherever you are. You will come to recognize growers, farmers and producers as you go week after week. Talk to them

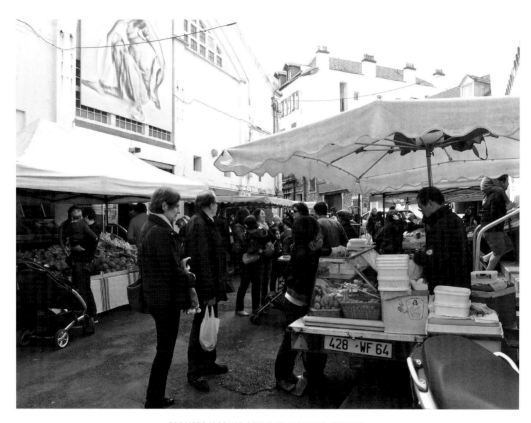

FARMERS MARKET SCENE IN BIARRITZ, FRANCE

and find out about the methods they use to grow and produce their products. Visit natural and organic food stores and get to know their mission statements, buying practices and community programs.

When I'm in New York City, I visit the Union Square farmers market on 14th Street, because I love the urban energy while still being able to mingle with, and buy from local growers from upstate New York and Long Island. When I'm in Boulder, Colorado, I shop at Alfalfa's, a neighborhood market owned by the "original" natural food entrepreneurs who remain true to their mission of supporting local organic and innovative food and wellness products. When I return to my roots on Long Island, Wild By Nature feels like home. I worked with its parent company, King Kullen, for almost 20 years, and together with Dana Conklin—a member of "the King's" founding family, realized her vision to create an organic and natural foods business.

The bottom line is that buying at farmers markets supports the environment and helps maintain open space for the local farm industry. And shopping at local and natural food markets makes it that much easier to find nutritional and artisanal products.

Turn weekends into a family activity to explore these markets, selecting food to experiment with for the week to come. It's a fun outing, and everyone will enjoy eating seasonal, pesticide-free food and properly fed and raised meat.

CHOOSE WHOLE FOODS

Europeans eat fewer processed foods. They know it's not as healthy as eating whole foods, because nutrients are lost in processing. Whole foods include fresh vegetables, fruits and whole-grains like whole-wheat, brown rice and oatmeal. For example, Europeans prefer to make fresh orange juice from real oranges. Jarred peanut butter is almost non-existent, because Europeans prefer to eat whole nuts. The selection of whole-grain breads in Europe is far more impressive than ours.

Bread has literally been the staff of life since pre-biblical times and maintains that status in European homes. Most families in France will have a freshly made baguette coming to their house that night for dinner—and it can often be seen sticking out of briefcases of men and women on their way home from work. Fresh bread is a staple in the household.

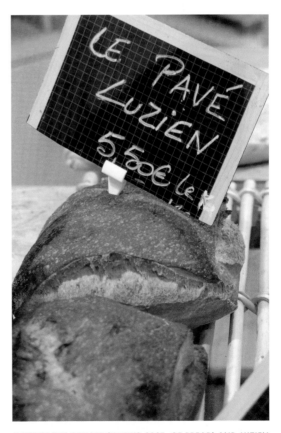

143

Europeans have done a great job in making bread healthy. They have so many more varieties of bread than we do: cereal, seeded, sourdough, quark, ancient grain, whole-wheat, corn, rye, spelt, olive, herb and the list goes on. Even individual towns may have their own specialty breads, using milled local grains or other innovations. Local artisanal bakers are a respected and important part of the community.

Sadly, Americans have really lowered the standard on what bread should look and taste like, or our current diet fads have turned it into public enemy #1. Today, the gluten-free craze is spreading: People suddenly believe that they shouldn't (for low-carb reasons) or can't

PAVE MEANS SQUARE (IN THIS CASE, OF BREAD) AND *LUZIEN* MEANS "SPECIALTY OF" SAINT-JEAN-DE-LUZ, FRANCE

(because of gluten or other intolerance issues) eat bread anymore. While celiac disease is a rare but serious immune disorder related to the protein in wheat and other grains, it strikes only about one percent of our population. And while it is right to stay away from the spongy, overprocessed, long-shelf-life packaged breads in the bread aisle, don't give it up when it's made the way it was intended to be made.

Have you ever looked at the ingredients label on a seemingly healthy loaf of pre-sliced supermarket bread that manages to sit on the shelf for a week and stay soft? I often wondered why there were so many ingredients on the list if it only takes flour, water, salt and yeast to make bread. When you visit a bakery, ask if the breads are "par baked" or made from scratch. "Par baking" is when the bread (or cake) is partially baked and then frozen, as we described earlier.

No doubt there are a number of superb artisanal bakeries in the U.S., but certainly not on every street corner like in France! My favorite Parisian bakery, Boulangerie Eric Kayser, recently opened in Manhattan, and according to Lou Ramirez, one of the U.S. owners, there are plans to expand across the country. Pepperidge Farm may soon have a run for its money!

When selecting pastas, cereals, rice and crackers, go for the whole-grain version—without added fat, sugar or salt. Don't believe the advertisements on the outside of the box that say made with whole-grains. Instead, read the ingredient list to make sure the product is truly made *with 100-percent whole-grains*—not white flour with a sprinkling of whole-grains, which is unfortunately how most "whole-grain" products are made. Remember, white flour and other refined grains lack fiber and important trace minerals.

The Whole Grains Council offers a stamp on products that deliver at least eight grams of whole grains per serving. Unfortunately, food companies pay to join this trade organization and not every company chooses to do so. Nothing trumps reading the ingredient label!

It is important to consume 25 to 38 grams of fiber per day. Choose cereals and whole-grains with at least three grams of fiber per serving. And unlike in Europe, serving sizes vary, so pay attention to the serving size on the nutrition facts labels.

Oats, oat bran and oatmeal contain soluble fiber known to lower cholesterol and maintain blood sugar control—when part of a healthy diet.

For those with gluten intolerance or celiac disease, include gluten-free grains like amaranth, buckwheat, corn, millet, oats, quinoa, rice, sorghum, teff and wild rice. Note that although oats are inherently gluten-free, they are often contaminated with wheat during growing or processing, so make sure the label says gluten-free oats.

Other ingredients that often replace wheat flour in baked goods include arrowroot, beans, chestnuts, potato, tapioca and soy. Understand that gluten-free products are not necessarily healthier. In fact, I've noticed that many of the gluten-free "health-food" bakery products are loaded with even more fat and sugar than conventionally baked goods.

The general rule is to increase your consumption of whole foods, especially vegetables and fruits. I am sure you've heard similar advice a thousand times, but it bears repeating again (and again and again). This will help displace some of the processed food in your diet and will actually make choosing healthy foods very simple.

Even better, there's no need to count calories, grams of fat, or carbs when selecting whole foods that are more a product of nature than a product of industry. When you eat less processed and packaged foods and buy bulk and natural foods, you can save time reading labels. And ultimately, it's more economical!

AISLE BY AISLE

Shopping a grocery store in the U.S. is like navigating a minefield of ads, tempting you to buy the latest profit-generating product. Grocers have spent years studying marketing and layout, and designing displays so that you will be tempted to buy more food than you need, and especially to buy the foods that are being displayed in their "end-cap" positions at the end of every aisle.

Ever notice that the milk is at the exact opposite corner of the entrance? That's because the grocer wants you to walk past all the enticements for products that you don't want or need. Milk has always been a household food staple.

Traditionally, supermarkets in our country stock 75 to 80 percent of the store with packaged goods, known as the "center store." The average supermarket stocks 30,000 to 40,000 unique items versus 18,000 items in European markets. Although the packaged goods category is slowly growing in Europe, more emphasis is on healthy, organic, private label, and specialty products.

You might have heard the phrase, "walk the perimeter of the store." That is because the aisles with the healthiest food in the grocery store are those that line the three sides of the building—fresh produce, dairy, bakery, deli, seafood and meats.

Our oversized supermarkets tend to narrow the choices of fruits and vegetables by stocking the most popular varieties and those that can be stored for longer periods. It's a different story when it comes to the cornucopia of chips and cookies, all with long shelf lives.

There's been no one to guide you through the process—until now. Let's go through the store, aisle by aisle, on making smart grocery store decisions. Depending on the store, each department can have a different delivery schedule; ask the department managers which days they get fresh food delivered, so you know when to shop!

PRODUCE

Get to know the produce manager and find out when they receive deliveries. They are a wealth of information when it comes to learning about fresh, local and organic produce.

Europeans dislike genetically modified food. When I lived in Europe, I didn't have to worry about having to discover whether or not I was consuming GMOs. The European Union (EU) has in place one of the strictest systems in the world regarding GMOs, requiring extensive testing, labeling and monitoring of agricultural products. Alas, it is not done in our country.

GMO is an organism with genetic material that has been altered in the laboratory through the transferring of a gene from one species to another species. The health consequences of this are debatable, but it is certainly not natural. Luckily, there are ways to avoid buying GMO foods.

That annoying sticker that seems to be on every piece of produce in American supermarkets is called a "PLU (Price Look-Up) Sticker." The bar code on the sticker is used at the checkout counter to scan the item for a price check. The sticker also has a 4- or 5-digit code that proves useful for the consumer. It tells us if the item is genetically modified. Here is how to fully decipher the code:

Conventionally grown, non-GMO produce has a 4-digit code. Genetically modified, conventional produce has a 5-digit code, beginning with the number 8. Organically grown produce also has a 5-digit code, beginning with the number 9. The good news is that if an item is organically grown, it's automatically non-GMO. For packaged goods, look for the third-party certification label, verifying that the product is non-GMO.

Fresh produce that is harvested and sold in the same season is tastier, more nutritious, and economical. For example, apples are crispiest in the fall, and stone fruits like peaches, apricots and

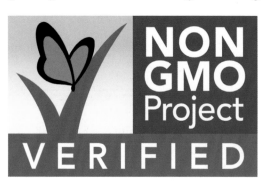

U.S. THIRD-PARTY LABEL TO VERIFY NON-GMO FOOD

146

nectarines are juiciest in the summer. Enjoy asparagus only in the spring. But carrots, potatoes and bananas can be enjoyed year-round.

Organically grown produce assures you that the farm did not use chemical pesticides, which has a positive environmental impact on land and water.

According to the Environmental Working Group (*www.ewg.org*), it's best to stick to organic when it comes to the "dirty dozen plus," which are fruits and vegetables with the highest pesticide residues. These are peaches, apples, sweet bell peppers, celery, nectarines (imported), strawberries, cherry tomatoes, grapes, spinach, hot peppers, cucumbers, potatoes, collard greens, kale, summer squash and zucchini.

The least contaminated, or "clean fifteen," items are onions, avocado, sweet corn, eggplant, sweet potatoes, pineapple, mango, grapefruit, asparagus, mushrooms, sweet peas (frozen), kiwi fruit, cantaloupe, cabbage and papaya. In the future, the sweet corn crop will be heavily sprayed, since pests are now invading even the GMO varieties. That's why it's always better to buy organically grown food.

No doubt, eating a variety of fruits and vegetables daily provides an abundance of vitamin A for healthy skin and eyes, along with vitamin C for healthy gums, skin and muscles, plus lowers risk for cancer and heart disease.

147

Sources of vitamin A include: apricots, cantaloupe, carrots, greens, romaine lettuce, pumpkin, sweet potatoes and spinach.

Sources of vitamin C include: kiwi, grapefruit, oranges, peaches, pineapples, plums, strawberries, broccoli, cabbage, cauliflower, corn, green beans, bell peppers, tomatoes and potatoes.

Fruits and vegetables are an excellent source of both soluble and insoluble fiber. Fiber is the roughage or what you do not absorb from plant-based foods. (Other high-fiber foods include: whole grains, legumes, cereals and nuts.)

An average pear contains two grams of soluble fiber
and two grams of insoluble fiber.

Soluble fiber is gummy and helps lower cholesterol and control blood sugar. Significant levels of soluble fiber are found in Brussels sprouts, okra, fresh artichoke and legumes (beans, peas and lentils).

Insoluble fiber is coarse and aids in digestion, prevents constipation and maintains the good bacteria in the colon. Significant levels of insoluble fiber are found in the tough skins of fruits and veggies.

*In addition to fruits and vegetables, dried beans, peas, wheat germ, brown rice,
barley, whole-grain pasta, whole-wheat couscous, dry-roasted and raw nuts
and seeds are all excellent sources of both soluble and insoluble fiber.*

Almost half of the fiber in fruit is found in the peel of a fruit, so eat your apples and pears with the peel on. To reduce exposure to pesticides, choose organically grown varieties when available.

Fruits and vegetables contain minerals and trace minerals. That's why it's better to eat whole fruits and vegetables rather than drink just the juice. Collard greens, kale, turnip greens, arugula, broccoli rabe, mustard greens, spinach, okra, oranges and broccoli contain a good dose of calcium.

For those looking for sources of iron, spinach and prunes are the best bets. Adding vitamin-C-rich foods to a meal, such as topping off spinach with tomato sauce, increases iron absorption. Cooking in a cast iron skillet is another way to increase iron consumption.

MEAT

If you care about where your meat comes from, how the animals were treated before slaughter, how they were fed, and if they were given antibiotics and hormones, then listen up! Marketers in the meat industry have invented some fancy names to convince you that conventional meat is as good as organic and grass-fed or pasture-raised meat. (As I discussed earlier, Europeans don't have these problems.)

"Grass-fed" is only used on meat labels from ruminant animals such as cattle and sheep, because they survive on grass. But some "grass-fed" herds are fed grains for a few months before being slaughtered. This results in fatter animals with more gut bacteria, including E. coli. The American Grassfed Association's certification program stipulates that animals can eat *only* grass, so look for this approval on labels. It's the gold standard!

"Pastured" means animals are outside eating grass but are also fed grains. That's because pigs, turkeys and chickens need more than grass to survive.

"Free-range" is a vague term used for poultry. Free-range is not foolproof, because chickens can be crammed in a barn and then let out to a feces-ridden concrete pen. This is hardly "free-range!"

Other certifications to look for are "Certified Humane Raised and Handled," "Animal Welfare Approved" and "USDA Organic." The ideal solution is to know the farmer and his or her farming practices.

While I don't recommend a Flintstones-size hunk of meat that takes up your whole plate, an occasional modest serving of high-quality extra-lean steak is fine for meat-lovers. Choose an extra-lean cut of grass-fed, organic beef and a grade of "Choice," or "Select." Do not buy "Prime," which contains the most marbled fat. Before cooking, trim away any visible fat.

Extra-lean beef contains less than five grams of total fat,
less than two grams of saturated fat and less than 95 milligrams of
cholesterol per three-and-a-half ounce serving (about 100 grams).

The following cuts are considered *extra-lean* and listed from most lean to least lean: eye-of-round roast or steak, sirloin tip side steak, top round roast or steak, bottom round roast or steak and top sirloin steak. When choosing ground meat, opt for organically raised, ground chicken or turkey breast. Make sure it's *only* the breast meat, and not ground with bones and skin—a common practice. The leanest poultry is the breast meat without the skin.

Pork tenderloin is the leanest cut of pork and is similar in calories and just slightly higher in fat than chicken breast. Whether pork or lamb, the lean cuts include tender-loin, loin chops and leg. Always buy your pork and lamb from local farmers who are known to practice high standards.

And when in doubt about what to buy, ask your butcher for advice.

SEAFOOD TWICE A WEEK

Europeans eat seafood when they are by the sea, and lake fish when they are by the lake. Most of the organic farmed fish from Northern Europe (not too far away) are tended with care so as not to harm the wild fish. Talk to your seafood retailer about your interest in shopping for sustainable and local fish, and find out which fish are wild but not endangered. If farmed, check that the fish was raised in an environmentally sensitive, sustainable way. The following website is a reputable reference for making responsible seafood choices based on where you live: *http://www.montereybayaquarium .org* (See Appendix for Seafood Watch.)

Pregnant and breast-feeding women are told to avoid certain fish high in methyl-mercury, PCBs (polychlorinated biphenyls) and other environmental contaminants so as not to damage their babies' developing nervous systems. Everyone should limit

149

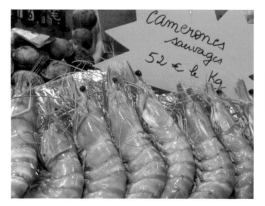
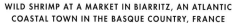
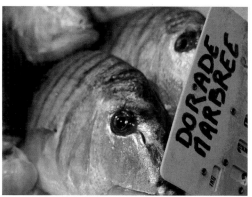

WILD SHRIMP AT A MARKET IN BIARRITZ, AN ATLANTIC COASTAL TOWN IN THE BASQUE COUNTRY, FRANCE

WILD DORADO (FISH) AT A MARKET IN BIARRITZ, AN ATLANTIC COASTAL TOWN IN THE BASQUE COUNTRY, FRANCE

fish high in these contaminants such as king mackerel, shark, swordfish, tilefish (aka golden bass or golden snapper), orange roughy and albacore tuna.

It's hard to balance concerns about heart health (which equates to choosing fish high in omega-3 fatty acids), environmental issues and mercury levels. There is no one single guide, but here are ten good choices including wild and farmed varieties that fit the bill: Wild Alaskan salmon, farmed Arctic char, Atlantic mackerel, sardines, Alaskan or British Columbia black cod (aka sablefish), anchovies, farmed oysters, farmed rainbow trout (aka golden trout), farmed mussels and Pacific halibut.

When buying canned fish, choose a brand that is packed in water, so you do not lose the natural omega-3s to the packed oil. If you opt for frozen, make sure there are no preservatives. (Read the ingredient label.) Young children should eat smaller portions of seafood: no more than three ounces for an average meal.

When cooking fish, don't fry it. You lose the heart-healthy, beneficial omega-3 fatty acids and raise the calories significantly! When using cooking oil made from polyunsaturated fat, do not heat it to a high temperature; this causes it to form potentially harmful compounds, especially when the oil is reused, which is a common practice in restaurants. And many restaurants still fry with partially hydrogenated oil—a source of trans fat, which has an adverse effect on cholesterol. Olive oil is good for sautéing. Compared to other cooking oils, it's fairly resistant to oxidative damage from heating.

DAIRY: AT LEAST THREE TIMES A DAY

Dairy is a staple in the Swiss, Italian and French diets and provides a significant amount of protein, vitamins A, D and calcium. Calcium is important for building and rebuilding healthy bones, teeth, and preventing osteoporosis. Vitamin D is important for calcium absorption. Dietary sources of Vitamin D are fish, whole eggs and fortified milk.

Women need between 1,200 to 1,500 milligrams of calcium daily, or four to five servings. An eight-ounce glass of milk has 300 milligrams of calcium. Buy fat-free or low-fat milk. Yogurt has the same amount of calcium in an eight-ounce serving; again, choose fat-free or low-fat varieties.

When available, choose low-fat or reduced-fat natural cheeses like Jarlsberg lite and Cabot's light cheddar. Ideally, look for three to five grams of fat or less per one-ounce serving. These types of cheeses are also good sources of calcium, with one-ounce averaging 200 milligrams.

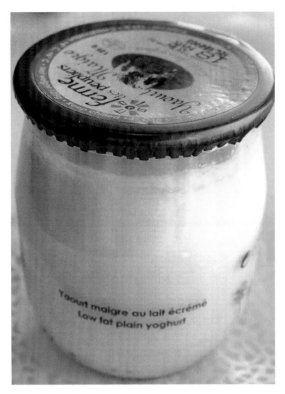

LOW-FAT YOGURT FROM NORMANDY, FRANCE

Fresh cheeses like ricotta, mozzarella, cottage, farmer, quark and feta tend to be lower in sodium and are also excellent sources of calcium. Buy low-fat or part-skim varieties.

Remember to choose rBGH-free dairy products. Choosing organic dairy automatically protects you from unwanted, added hormones and antibiotics.

BECOME A FRESH-AND-HEALTHY-FOOD ADVOCATE

Talk to the department managers who are involved in ordering foods for your supermarket. I can tell you from experience, having worked as a director for a supermarket chain for nearly 20 years, that they do listen. Comment cards are read at weekly meetings. Supermarkets want to please their customers by giving you the foods and services that you want. If you let them hear your voice, you can make a difference!

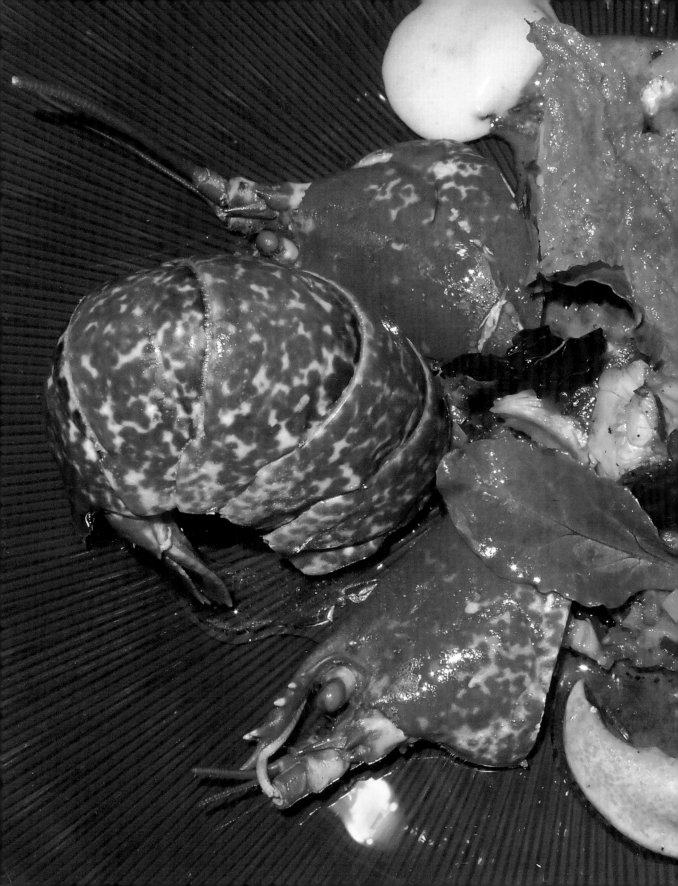

Chapter 9

DINE OUT BOLDLY

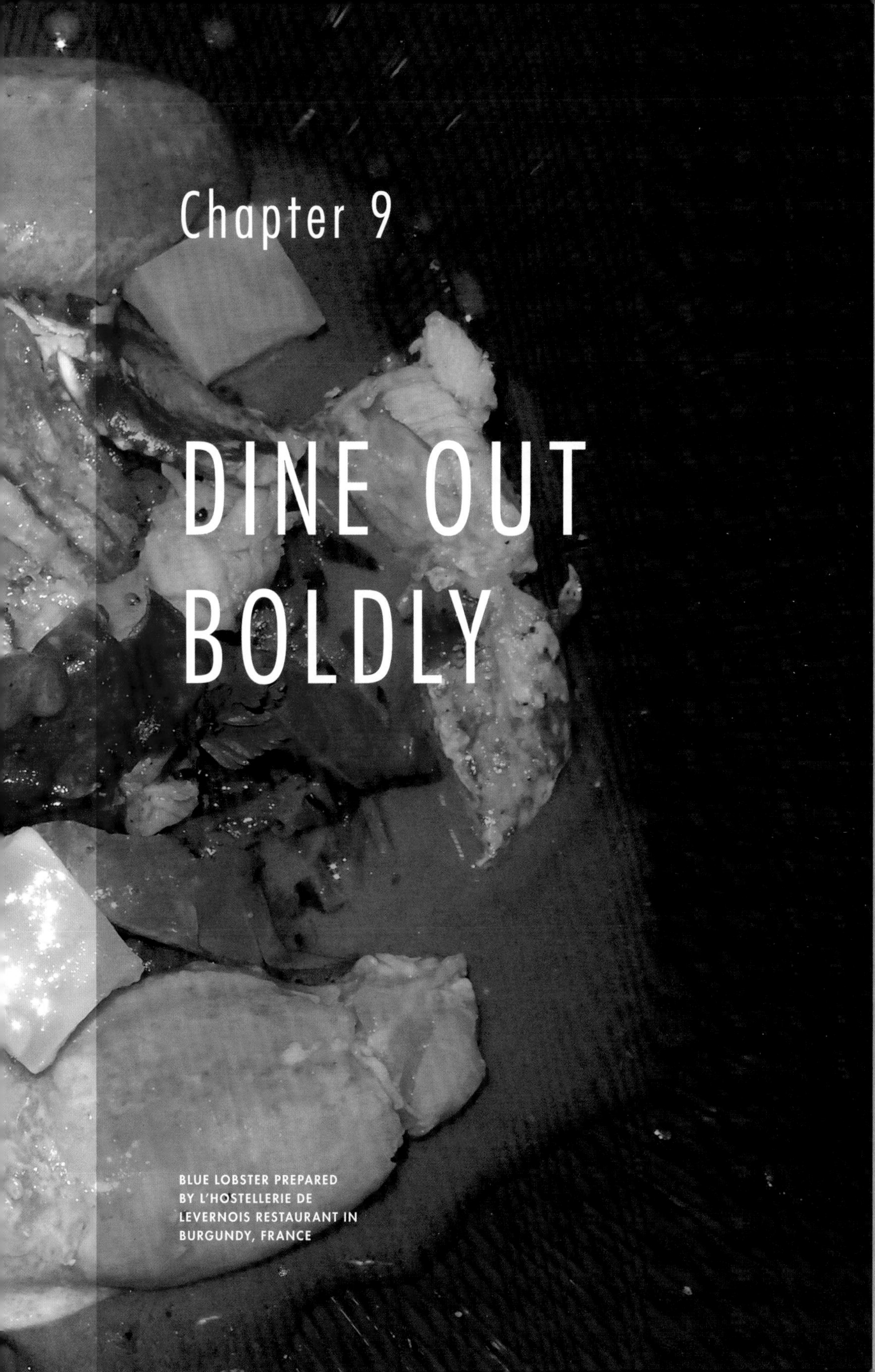

BLUE LOBSTER PREPARED
BY L'HOSTELLERIE DE
LEVERNOIS RESTAURANT IN
BURGUNDY, FRANCE

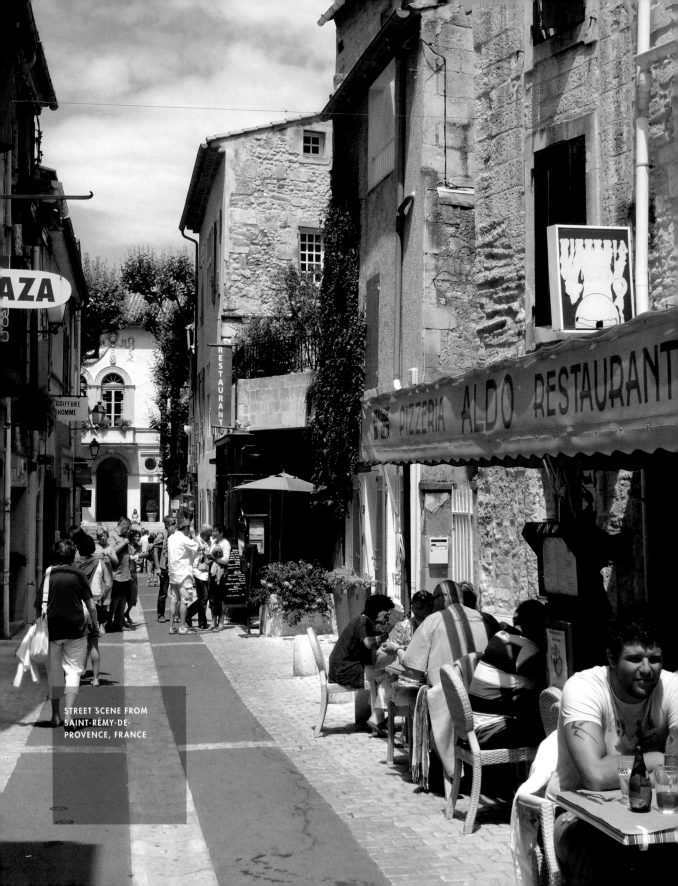

STREET SCENE FROM
SAINT-RÉMY-DE-
PROVENCE, FRANCE

O h, how I enjoyed eating my way through Europe, with an eye on nutrition and a mission to figure out just how Europeans seem to feast for hours at a restaurant and remain slender and healthy.

With many European countries being just a train ride away from Switzerland, it was easy to explore the eateries of Italy and France. I delved into menus and met chefs that I'd only ever dreamed about meeting. While this sounds like an easy recipe for weight gain, I was able to stay slim, delight in every bite, and get the scoop on European secrets of dining out well!

The French, Swiss and Italians treat eating out as a special occasion, not just an opportunity to chow down. Dining is not only about eating: It's also about manners, conversation and living in the moment. Instinctively, Europeans seem able to balance enjoying themselves with maintaining self-control. They don't overstuff themselves or, as we know it, "pig out."

In contrast, the American appetite seems insatiable. We eat out often and prefer large portions of everything, even diet soda! According to the National Restaurant Association, nearly half our food budget is spent on restaurant food. Studies show that eating out just one meal a week could equal a two-pound weight gain per year. Take a look at the menus and portion sizes, and you'll see why!

Diet drinks are unhealthy and do not help you lose weight.

This chapter will explore just how to find the right balance of enjoyment and discipline while eating out anywhere, whether you're in Chicago, Illinois, or Lyon, France.

PLAN YOUR DINING EXPERIENCE

European restaurants are not open 24 hours a day, seven days a week like ours are. They keep specific business hours for meal times. Many are closed on Saturday nights, which we consider "date night." And generally speaking, eating out is more expensive in Europe, compared to the U.S., so Europeans eat at home more often than they dine out, and meal times are, for the most part, consistent.

We Americans are pretty spoiled: Our lifestyle tends to include a multitude of 24/7, reasonably priced, dining options. But the ability to eat out whenever we want, tempts us to overindulge at any given moment.

Knowing you're limited as to when you can dine out makes the experience much more special. Planning when and where you'll go and what you'll order ahead of time are some of the best "behavior modification" techniques you can use to lose weight. The thought we put into meal planning will make us less likely to eat impulsively.

When you're in Europe, with its restricted times to eat out, you learn to plan ahead. My husband and I once went hiking in the mountains of Switzerland and lost track of time. Around lunchtime, we realized that the only restaurant nearby, a café, was about to close, and we were still two miles from the village. We had eaten no food for hours, so my husband ran ahead to order us food before the café, the only place for miles, closed down.

To my relief, when I finally arrived at the cafe, there was a small lunch waiting for me: a cold plate with a leaf of lettuce, two slices of cheese and bread. While it wasn't exactly what I had been dreaming about during my six-mile hike, at least we were fed. We learned a valuable lesson from that experience: Always find out the opening and closing times of restaurants in the area we'll be visiting.

Let's face it: There are occasions when you must be spontaneous, so if you can't find a restaurant open when you need one, search out ethnic options like Chinese, Indian or Middle Eastern. Hard-working immigrants often keep their restaurants open more often and for longer hours.

Also, check out the areas around farmers markets and shopping malls. Cafés and diners are likely to be open because of the increased foot traffic on the weekends. Another option is to plan ahead and bring along a picnic lunch to eat outdoors, weather permitting.

*Plan ahead, make restaurant reservations, and map out your day
so that meals are part of the schedule.*

Making restaurant reservations is always wise. If you are eating casually, research your options so you don't end up at a fast food drive-in! Keep a food diary to remind you when you're likely to be hungry. It helps you decide when to plan your dining-out activities.

Choose the desired location and do a "Google" search on dining options in that area. For restaurant recommendations, reviews and reservations in the U.S., I often use *opentable.com, seamless.com, urbanspoon.com, tripadvisor.com, zagat.com, happycow.net and yelp.com.* Once you narrow down the choices, you can also visit the restaurants' websites directly to view their menus ahead of time.

Restaurant chains often provide nutritional information on their websites, so you can decide whether the menu is right for your dietary needs.

HELP YOUR SERVER HELP YOU

Whether in Europe or the U.S., there are vast differences, both in what restaurants serve and in how they run their establishments. Service can vary widely, from making sure you get exactly what you want to offering a minimum amount of help, as in the case of a server handing you an "Ipad" to place your own order.

The French are extremely proud of their cuisine, and waiters may either help you fully appreciate the meal by offering eloquent explanations of menu items, or have a superior attitude and tell you that the chef permits no changes or special requests.

On the other hand, Italians are warm and expressive, and make you feel like part of the family. By nature, Italian servers will likely be helpful in attending to your dietary concerns.

The Swiss may not seem as warm and friendly; however, it's just that they have a more formal attitude and are often less flexible in accepting changes to the set menu.

Thus, if you're not getting the service you deserve, feel free to request another server who is more willing to address your concerns.

Establishing rapport between you and your server is key to maximizing your dining-out experience. Don't be shy. Feel confident in communicating your needs and fully understand your options. This will allow you to make smart decisions about how much and what to order. The server is your link to the chef or cook, so if you're friendly and inquisitive, you're more likely to get what you want.

Read your menu carefully, listen to the specials, and when your server is ready to take the order, ask any questions you wish about the ingredients and preparation of the selections that appeal to you. Remember, you're paying for the meal, so you have a right to ask for modifications to the dishes you order. You may not get all of them, but nothing ventured, nothing gained. Right?

Be assertive when you're ordering in a restaurant.

Ask the waiter and the chef to take an extra step like putting the sauce on the side of your dish or substituting whole-wheat pasta for white pasta. The owners of the restaurant want you to come back and be a loyal patron.

THE TABLE IS YOURS, SO FEEL FREE TO LINGER

The wonderful part about dining out in Europe is that you feel as though you can stay for as long as you want. There's no pressure to leave so that someone else can take

157

your table. Restaurants there never expect diners to rush through a meal, and would consider it rude to hover around the table waiting for the check to be paid. In fact, the restaurant industry is less profitable in Europe, because the American practice of maximizing table turnover is almost non-existent.

Contrast that with America: Often, I've called for a 7 p.m. reservation at certain popular restaurants in New York, only to be told I can have the table if I understand that I have to vacate it for the 9 p.m. reservation. That simply wouldn't happen in Europe.

Wherever you are dining, give yourself at least one hour to finish your meal, which is good for digestion while fitting into our busy "American" lifestyle!

As an added benefit, your lack of stress over giving up your table is actually good for you; statistics show that people who linger at the dinner table tend *not* to be overweight. Why? Well, it takes roughly 20 minutes for the stomach and brain to register fullness, and most of us are finished eating in 10 minutes once the food arrives. Then we're on to the next serving. But since our stomachs haven't communicated with our brains yet, by the time we've reached 20 minutes, we've eaten far too much and feel overstuffed and overstretched!

For a casual meal out, plan to linger for at least one hour.
For more formal dining or with larger groups, allow two to three hours.

Allotting at least one hour for a casual meal will give you enough time to be seated, speak with your server and fellow guests, enjoy the food, and digest it properly.

TAKE A WALK BEFORE AND AFTER DINNER

Sure, you're not in Paris. You may be in a strip mall in the suburbs of Minnesota on a cold winter's night, but try to follow the European habit of taking a stroll to burn calories after a meal. This helps reduce blood sugar and speeds up metabolism. Europeans even stroll in the cold, so bundle up and enjoy an invigorating walk!

You can also walk before dinner in daylight to receive some natural vitamin D from the sun. Remember we need 15 minutes a day. When traveling by car, park a distance from the restaurant so you can build up an appetite on the walk over and burn extra calories after the meal by walking back to the car.

To further boost calorie-burning, stay away from the sofa and TV, and engage in some yoga, bowling or dancing. And then relax over a candlelit dinner!

CONSIDER OPTING FOR APPETIZERS

A popular trend in many European restaurants is creating a meal of small dishes known as *tapas* in Spain, otherwise known as a "tasting menu" in France. These small dishes are indeed quite small, so even if you linger for hours, enjoying one plate after another, you're not eating more food, but you are adding new, palate-pleasing foods to your repertoire. The small portions allow you to enjoy new dishes without overwhelming your taste buds with too much of one thing. Instead, your palate is stimulated by multiple tastes and flavors.

Eating a variety of new tastes actually decreases your need to eat too much. It also removes any obligation you might feel to eat a single dish you may not really enjoy. As we Americans are card-carrying members of the "Clean Your Plate" club, when the menu offers oversized restaurant portion, choosing appetizer portions can help you avoid overeating.

Instead of ordering an appetizer and an entrée, order two appetizers, or order one appetizer and share an entrée with a friend—or take half home.

In order to set up your own "Super-Healthy Plate," choose at least one vegetable-based appetizer, such as minestrone soup or a beet salad with dressing on the side. Always order an extra side of steamed, seasonal veggies, and you might, like me, ask for tomato or marinara sauce for those freshly steamed veggies.

THINK "MODEST" WHEN YOU THINK DESSERT

If you look at desserts at an American restaurant, they are often a gut-busting size and oozing with calories, fat and sugar. Do these desserts sound familiar: chocolate lava cake, banana split, or bourbon pecan pie?

In France, people opt for a bite-size sampling of dessert called petits fours, a miniature confection usually served with coffee. Italians enjoy a biscotto, a small but flavorful biscuit, with wine at the end of the meal. The Swiss are usually happy with a zesty piece of cheese and dried fruit to end a meal.

The good news is, you have many options available here in the United States. You can share a dessert four ways, opt for a scoop of sorbet, bowl of berries, poached pear, or share a fruit-filled meringue. Meringue is a popular Swiss and French

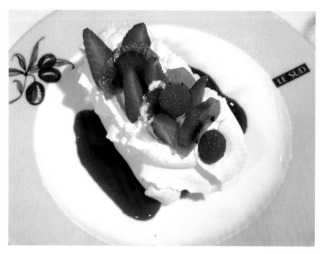

FRUIT-FILLED MERINGUE AT LE SUD RESTAURANT IN LYON, FRANCE

dessert made with egg whites and sugar. Otherwise, wait until you get home and enjoy a healthy, homemade dessert, such as yogurt with fresh fruit, a sliver of low-fat cheese with a sliced apple, or a modest slice of homemade apple cake. (See Chapter 14 for mouthwatering dessert recipes.)

Alternatively, take a stroll to your favorite frozen yogurt shop and try a four-ounce serving of tart yogurt, topped with fresh fruit. If it's cold outside, have a hot chocolate made with fat-free or low-fat milk instead!

Try to think of dessert as "a taste of something rich and delicious," like a spoonful of your friend's rich chocolate cake, rather than something that might fill your entire plate and will definitely expand your waistline. If you desire a larger dessert, ask for your favorite fruit, either cooked, dried or fresh, as a sweet ending to a meal.

Just a reminder—one serving of a typical American restaurant chain's brownie can have as many as 1,600 calories and 77 grams of fat. Yikes! It will add an instant half pound of fat to your body. Now, seriously, is it worth it?

PREPARE YOUR FAVORITE RESTAURANT DISHES AT HOME

To re-create the restaurant experience at home, take a dish you love from your favorite restaurant and experiment with making a healthier version of it. That way you can control the ingredients, which is often what you cannot control at restaurants.

When I was consulting for a major supermarket chain, I was continually testing new recipes, and my sons were the taste-testers. My kids love cheesecake, but I couldn't bear to watch them eat spoonfuls of artery-clogging cream cheese and sugar. The average cheesecake recipe has two pounds of cream cheese in it, not to mention a lot of butter for the graham cracker crust.

I knew I could find an alternative when I saw they enjoyed Italian cheesecake as much as American cheesecake. American cheesecake is made with processed cream cheese, while Italian cheesecake is made with fresh ricotta cheese and is

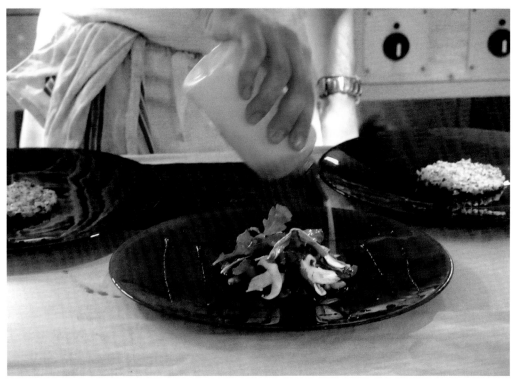

SAUCE POURED AT THE BOTTOM OF THE PLATE AT L'HOSTELLERIE DE LEVERNOIS RESTAURANT IN BURGUNDY, FRANCE

The French make wonderful roast meats, too. Choose a lean variety, like Cornish hen, or medallions of pork—typically from pork loin.

One of my favorite traditional French dishes is *ratatouille,* a vegetable dish made of tomatoes, eggplant, peppers, onions, summer squash and a bit of olive oil.

The French love sauces, so ask for them to be served on the side so you can control how much you use.

In France, sauce is served on the bottom of the plate so you can regulate how much you eat with your food.

French enjoy salads, and you can't do better than a classic Salad Niçoise. I don't like anchovies, so I also ask that they "hold" the anchovies and serve the dressing on the side.

For dessert, choose a poached pear or share a fruit crêpe. Remember, you only need a few yummy bites!

Chinese Restaurants—Chinese food is covered in oil, cornstarch and salty sauce loaded with MSG (monosodium glutamate). So order dishes with your favorite vegetables, steamed with sauces served on the side. Sweet and sour sauce is your best bet for a dipping sauce because it's lowest in fat and salt (it contains sugar). If you must choose one dish, opt for *Moo Goo Gai Pan*. It's typically made with chicken, mushrooms, water chestnuts and bok choy. The sauce consists of oil, broth, soy sauce, oyster sauce, cornstarch, MSG and sometimes sugar. Still ask for no MSG and as little oil and sauce as possible. Steamed vegetable dumplings are also a good option.

In Chinese restaurants in the U.S., brown rice is typically available as a healthier alternative to white rice—it's higher in fiber, trace minerals and vitamin E.

As to dessert, feel free to indulge in a fortune cookie: It's only about 30 calories!

Greek Restaurants—Although Greek cuisine is generally healthy, be aware of some potential pitfalls. Gyros are Greek hero sandwiches—beef or lamb stuffed into a large pita—with sauce dripping from the sides. These can add up to 800 calories. You should also avoid falafels—the chickpea balls are deep-fried.

Instead, choose a Greek salad (light on the feta cheese with dressing on the side), hummus with pita bread, or stuffed grape leaves to start. The tart yogurt-and-cucumber sauce (tzatziki) goes nicely with roasted or grilled chicken, lamb or fish. Chicken or fish kebobs are the leanest option.

The multi-layered dessert, *baklava*, is made with honey, nuts and buttery pastry. An average serving is 550 calories, so be sure to share it four ways!

Indian Restaurants—Indian restaurants always have vegetarian options; most are non-vegan. Beware of creamy curries, buttery naan breads and fried samosas. *Malai* is cream, and *ghee* is clarified butter; both fats are widely used in Indian cooking.

Start with lentil soup, and then choose a low-calorie option such as *tandoori* chicken or fish. "Tandoori" means the meat, fish or veggie is marinated in yogurt and spices, and then cooked in a high-heat clay oven or tandoor. Go easy on the breads, avoid the stuffed ones, and asked for a baked—not fried—roti instead.

Other foods to try are *paneer* (mild, fresh cheese), *raita sauce* (made from yogurt) and *yellow lentils*.

Italian Restaurants—Typically, Italian restaurants use olive oil instead of butter, and although olive oil is as high in calories as butter—both are 100-percent fat—it is a source of monounsaturated fat and therefore healthier for your heart. Since it is high in calories, ask that the chef use as little as possible.

Italian salads are usually an assortment of fresh lettuces and seasonal vegetables, from arugula, endive, radicchio and fennel to artichoke, mushroom, tomato and green beans. Add freshly shaved Parmesan cheese and a squeeze of lemon; these are sure to satisfy any salad connoisseur!

Other healthy starters include steamed mussels and soups, like tomato-based minestrone, or *pasta fagiole* (pasta with beans).

For entrees, share *chicken cacciatore* (chicken in a tomato-based sauce) and *gnocchi* (a dumpling made with potato, ricotta cheese, egg and semolina flour) in a marinara sauce. For a lighter meal, dig in to a half order of whole-wheat pasta with marinara or red clam sauce and request a serving of steamed broccoli rabe. Freshly grated Parmesan cheese rules over powdered, often "counterfeit," Parmesan.

Lobster Fra Diavolo is lobster in a spicy tomato sauce served over linguine and is usually enough for two to share. Shrimp marinara is a low-calorie choice so long as they don't fry the shrimp.

Want pizza? Ask for a vegetarian pizza with fresh mozzarella or no cheese—or remove half the cheese. Avoid fried foods like fried calamari or zucchini, buttery garlic bread, and the overly cheesy lasagna and creamy pasta with Alfredo sauce.

Italians are generous and serve large portions, so consider ordering a salad, then share an additional starter and an entrée.

Japanese Restaurants—It's no accident that the Japanese have one of the highest life-expectancy rates, thanks to their healthy diets of fish, rice and fresh vegetables. Unfortunately, their high stomach cancer rates are linked to Japan's high-sodium diets.

Start with a miso soup or a salad; Japanese dressings are ginger-based and typically made without added fats. Teriyaki chicken, beef or salmon are good, low-fat choices, but the teriyaki sauce is high in salt, so ask for it on the side.

Eat sushi if the seafood is fresh and sustainable. You can create your own rolls, so choose ingredients such as cooked shrimp, real crab, brown rice, asparagus, cucumber, avocado and squash. You can also request the rolls to be made with less or no rice, and some restaurants offer brown rice for a small up-charge. Brown rice is a whole-grain, high in fiber and nutrition. Request spicy rolls made without mayonnaise. Ask for low-sodium soy sauce and use it sparingly. If fresh wasabi is an option, go for it!

Beware of the seaweed salads; many are colored with green dye! Choose hijiki, which is pure black seaweed. Avoid pink ginger, because the pink color is from artificial dye. Ginger should be white.

Skip the deep-fried tempura and fried ice cream. On special occasions, share a red bean mochi ice cream. This is red bean ice cream encased in a rice flour shell, made from boiled rice flour. Fat and calories vary according to the size of the mochi, so be aware of portion size and share.

Mexican Restaurants—For starters, try the cold tomato soup called *gazpacho* (originally from Spain), but avoid the fried nacho chips for obvious reasons.

For an entrée, order the grilled chicken, shrimp or vegetable fajitas, and ask for soft baked tortillas. Or try a fish taco with salsa and request a soft shell instead of the crispy fried one. Choose guacamole made from avocado—a nutritious "good" fat, as a dip, instead of heaps of cheddar cheese and sour cream. Steer clear of the high-calorie taco salads, cheesy enchiladas and gut-busting burritos.

American Restaurants—This applies to diners, burger joints, delis and steak houses. If you're going to get a burger, opt for a veggie, salmon, tuna, buffalo or bison burger. Make sure the veggie burger is not fried, and if you prefer a turkey burger, be sure it's made from turkey breast, without skin and bones.

If you must have a steak, order a lean cut like London broil, or share one with a friend. Then, if you and a friend each order a baked potato to go with your shared steak, you'll have a full meal. My favorite diner food is a veggie egg-white omelet with a baked sweet potato. Fresh fruit or a side salad is a good substitute for those tempting, fat-laden French fries. (Home fries are *usually* less fatty than French fries.)

Recently, as a trend to offering healthier options at fast food restaurants, wraps and egg-white sandwiches are advertised as good-for-you breakfast and lighter-lunch alternatives. Although they carry lower caloric loads than traditional breakfast and lunch fare, and advertisements use words like cage-free eggs and whole-grain bread, most are full of additives and preservatives. While the wraps and breads may contain a small amount of whole grain, hydrogenated fat and dough softeners are typically added to extend the shelf life. Even the egg whites are often mixed with poor quality oils, starches and fillers.

At a deli, be prepared for oversized sandwiches. A big, thick American sandwich can have six to nine ounces of meat, whereas you want about half that amount—like a European. Take the other half home for tomorrow's lunch.

Whatever the venue, if the portion is large, remember that you can always ask for a doggie bag to carry out! Even better, ask your server to bring a container before you begin to eat. Wrapping up the excess when it arrives prevents you from eating more than you should. And wrapping up your own leftovers means fewer food handlers and less risk of contamination.

Some restaurants (especially hotels) offer child-sized portions of what you want, which is more likely to be the proper, healthful size. The sad truth is that many children's menu choices, like macaroni and cheese, hot dogs, French fries, fried chicken nuggets, are often loaded with more fat and salt than adult menu choices.

Better yet, let's now stay home, head for the kitchen, and create a delicious meal from the super-healthy recipes in Part Three!

Baby Moon RESTAURANT SINCE 1970

On the LOW FAT SIDE and LOW CARB Choices*

Salad Pizza: Chopped Salad Greens on Whole Wheat Crust
Per Slice: Calories: 220 Fat: 8g Cholesterol: 0mg

Vegetable Pizza: with FAT FREE MOZZARELLA
Per Slice: Calories: 220 Fat: 2g Cholesterol: 10mg

Chopped Salad: Arugula, Endive, Radicchio, Tomato, Red Pepper, Red Onion, Walnuts, FAT FREE MOZZARELLA and Special FAT FREE Balsamic Dressing
Calories: 220 Fat: 8g Cholesterol: 0mg

*Low Carb Grilled Chicken Parmigiana with FAT FREE MOZZARELLA Served with a Steamed Vegetable
Calories: 300 Fat: 4g Cholesterol: 95mg Total Carbs: 17g Dietary Fiber: 4g Effective Net Carbs: 13g

Baked Ziti with FAT FREE MOZZARELLA Over Steamed Spinach with Tomato Basil Sauce
Calories: 515 Fat: 3g Cholesterol: 10mg

Brown Rice Penne (wheat free) with Turkey Meatballs Over Steamed Escarole, Tomato Basil Sauce
Calories: 445 Fat: 3g Cholesterol: 95mg

Baked Eggplant with Pasta and Tomato Basil Sauce
Calories: 255 Fat: 1g Cholesterol: 0mg

Grilled Vegetable Platter & Cannellini Beans
Calories: 340 Fat: 2g Cholesterol: 0mg

Whole Wheat Pasta, Beans, Fresh Vegetables with Tomato Basil Sauce
Calories: 450 Fat: 2g Cholesterol: 0mg

Pasta Delicata: Linguini with Spinach, Sun-Dried Tomatoes and Grilled Chicken
Calories: 525 Fat: 3g Cholesterol: 70mg

Grilled Lemon Chicken topped with Chopped Salad Served with a Steamed Vegetable & Pasta with a Tomato Basil Sauce
Calories: 390 Fat: 3g Cholesterol: 95mg

Flounder "Light Anesca": Baked with Fresh Tomatoes and a touch of Capers Served with Steamed Vegetables & Pasta with a Tomato Basil Sauce
Calories: 440 Fat: 3g Cholesterol: 100mg

Roasted Balsamic Salmon with Fresh Tomato and Spring Mix Salad
Calories: 360 Fat: 18g Cholesterol: 100mg

Salmon contains beneficial Omega 3 Fats. The American Heart Association recommends two servings of fish weekly, particularly fish high in Omega 3 Fatty Acids, such as Salmon. This entree is NOT low fat.

Cappuccino with FAT FREE MILK
Calories: 40 Fat: 0g Cholesterol: 2mg

Consulting Nutritionist: Layne Lieberman, RD, MS, CDN
Portion Size may Vary-Please use your Best Judgement. UPON REQUEST, NO SALT WILL BE ADDED

167

LAYNE'S MENU HELPS PATRONS CHOOSE HEALTHY OPTIONS, AT BABY MOON RESTAURANT, WESTHAMPTON BEACH, NY

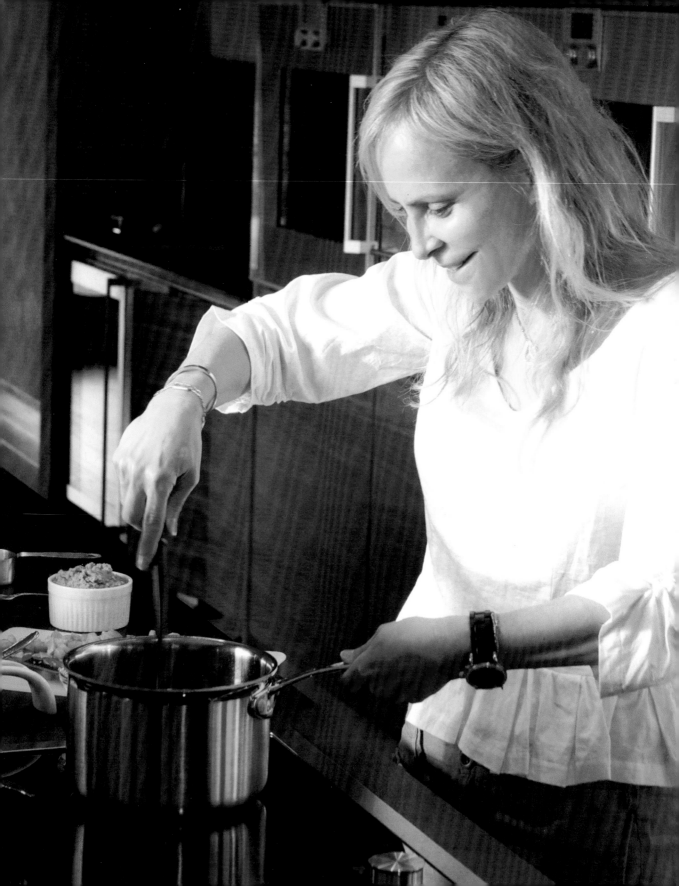

Part Three

RECIPES FOR A GUILT-FREE INDULGENCE

169

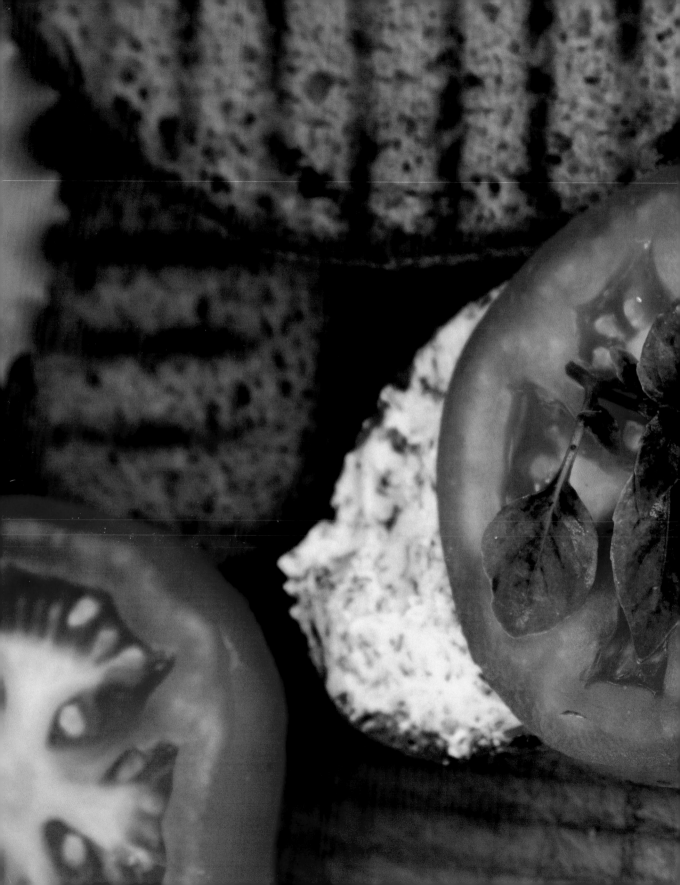

Chapter 10

BREAKFAST— LE PETIT DÉJEUNER

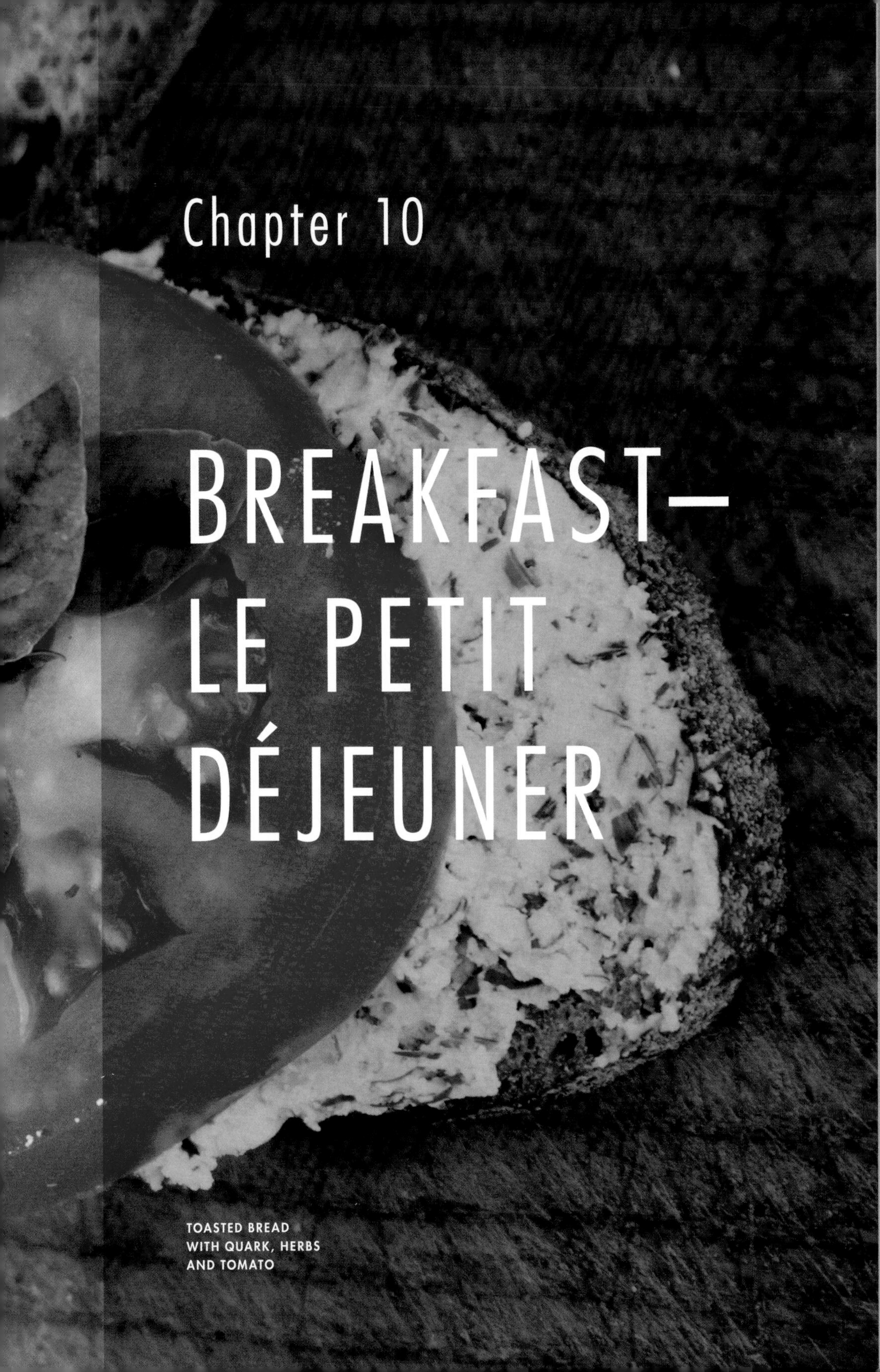

TOASTED BREAD
WITH QUARK, HERBS
AND TOMATO

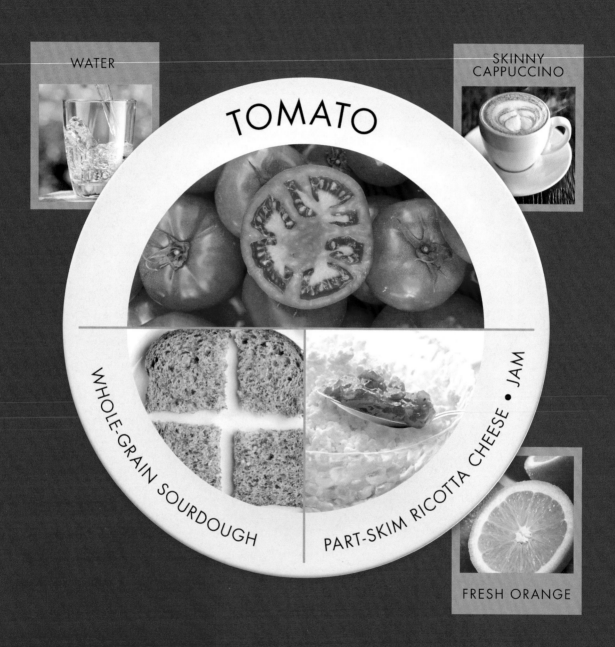

WATER

SKINNY CAPPUCCINO

TOMATO

WHOLE-GRAIN SOURDOUGH

PART-SKIM RICOTTA CHEESE • JAM

FRESH ORANGE

SUPER-HEALTHY BREAKFAST PLATE GUIDE

D id you ever realize that a "Continental breakfast," a basket of bread and pastries served with coffee, tea and fresh juice offered at hotels worldwide, is not for the purveyor to make extra money, but in fact comes from the European practice of eating a light breakfast?

Rather than overloading their plates with eggs and sausage, Europeans start the day on a lighter note, opting for coffee or tea, a small cup of juice from two fresh oranges and a slice of bread with jam. A splurge may be a sweet pastry instead of bread.

Americans are brought up to believe that a big breakfast is the most important meal of the day. While it's true that your body needs nourishment in the morning after a fast, it does not necessarily correlate to needing a large amount of food.

Europeans often joke about the Big American Breakfast, which is promoted as such in European restaurants, mostly for tourists. Meanwhile, we Americans are constantly being urged to eat bigger breakfasts. Food companies even hire nutritionists to send out the same message!

While breakfast is important, it's not as critical as we've been trained to believe. Breaking the fast *lightly* is the ideal approach. The following recipes offer a healthy twist on both traditional American and European favorites.

Although the listed ingredients of these recipes throughout Part Three do not specify brands, use organic and local ingredients whenever possible. Also keep in mind that when a recipe calls for an egg, assume it's a large egg, not a jumbo, and all vegetables and fruits are medium-sized, not supersized.

Temperature equivalents (U.S. standard to European metric):
212 degrees Fahrenheit equals 100 degrees Celsius (Boiling point)
250 degrees Fahrenheit equals 121 degrees Celsius
300 degrees Fahrenheit equals 149 degrees Celsius
350 degrees Fahrenheit equals 177 degrees Celsius
400 degrees Fahrenheit equals 205 degrees Celsius
450 degrees Fahrenheit equals 233 degrees Celsius
500 degrees Fahrenheit equals 260 degrees Celsius

BREAKFAST RECIPES

APPLE MANGO WITH YOGURT AND OATS

Serves 4

½ cup rolled oats
1 cup nonfat Greek vanilla yogurt
3 medium apples, cored and diced
1 mango, pitted, peeled and diced
½ teaspoon ground cinnamon

In a medium-sized bowl, combine oats with yogurt and set aside. Preheat oven to 350 degrees Fahrenheit. Place apples in a baking dish and bake for 15 to 20 minutes or until soft.

Add mango and cinnamon to the cooked apples and mix gently. Top the oat-yogurt mixture with fruit and serve.

If you prefer your oats on the soft side, prepare the oats and yogurt a day ahead of time. A batch lasts for three days in the fridge.

To save 15 minutes, microwave the apples instead of baking them. Place apples in a microwave-safe baking dish, then loosely cover dish with a dishtowel and microwave for 3 minutes, or until apples are soft and juicy. Follow remainder of recipe instructions.

Alternatively, use pears instead of apples and fold in any seasonal fresh fruit.

Per serving (255 grams): 188 calories, 0.9 grams fat, 38 milligrams sodium, 40 grams carbohydrate, 5.8 grams dietary fiber, 6.6 grams protein.

BIRCHER MUESLI

Serves 4

(Requires soaking overnight)
¾ cups rolled oats
1 cup fat-free milk or original almond milk
½ cup nonfat Greek vanilla yogurt
½ cup dates, chopped
1 apple, chopped
1 banana, diced
1 tablespoon fresh lemon juice
¼ cup sliced almonds, toasted (optional)

In a large bowl, prepare the muesli: mix oats, milk, yogurt and dates; cover and refrigerate overnight.

The next morning, in a medium bowl, combine the apple and banana (or whatever fruit you prefer) with the lemon juice.

Top muesli with the fruit mixture, sprinkle with optional toasted almonds and serve.

Vary the fruit topping according to the season. Stone fruit like apricots, plums, peaches and nectarines are seasonal summer fruits.

To lower carbohydrates and calories, use plain yogurt instead of vanilla.

Per serving with dates and almonds (212 grams): 248 calories, 4.2 grams fat, 46 milligrams sodium, 47.4 grams carbohydrate, 6.1 grams dietary fiber, 8.7 grams protein.

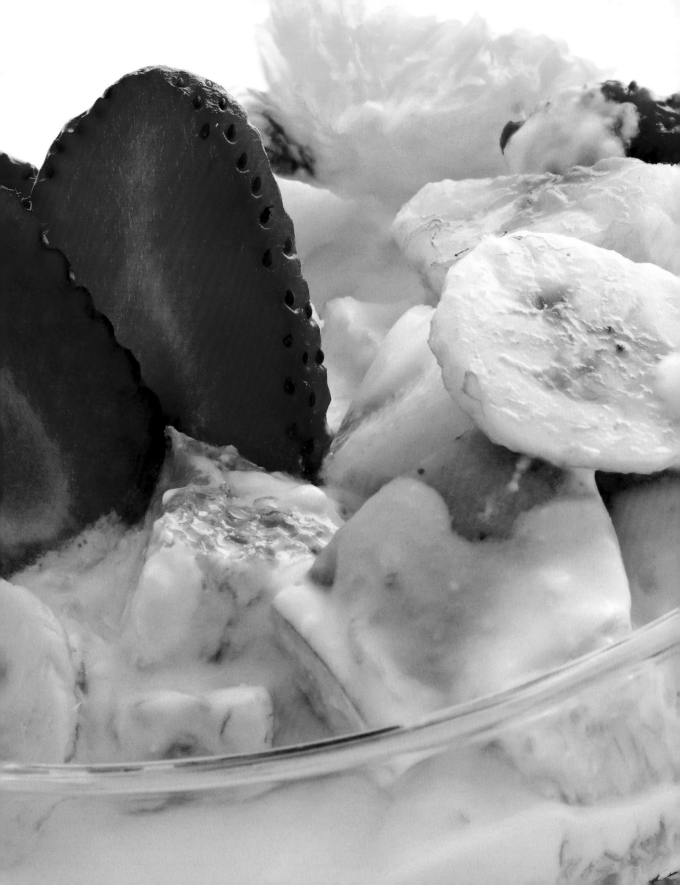

POLENTA GRITS WITH NUT BUTTER AND BANANA

Serves 2

1 cup water
1 cup fat-free milk or original almond milk
¼ teaspoon sea salt
½ cup stone-ground corn grits/polenta
1 ripe banana
1 tablespoon creamy natural almond butter (or creamy natural peanut butter, walnut butter, cashew butter or tahini)
¼ teaspoon pure vanilla extract

In a medium saucepan, bring water and milk to a low boil over medium heat. Stir in the salt and polenta; reduce heat to simmer. Cook polenta over low heat until thick and creamy, stirring often, about 10 minutes.

While the polenta cooks, in a small bowl, mash the banana with the nut butter and add vanilla extract. Spoon the polenta over the banana-almond butter mixture. Serve at any temperature.

For fewer calories and less fat, omit the nut butter and serve the polenta on top of a sliced banana.

Per serving with nut butter (345 grams): 278 calories, 4.8 grams fat, 290 milligrams sodium, 48 grams carbohydrate, 3.8 grams dietary fiber, 9.5 grams protein.

GOLDEN BREAD (AKA FRENCH TOAST)

Serves 6

6 slices bread (preferably whole-grain)
2 eggs plus 2 egg whites, lightly beaten
1 teaspoon vanilla extract
½ cup fat-free milk or original almond milk
1 teaspoon ground cinnamon
Nonstick cooking spray, olive oil

In a large, shallow, flat-bottom bowl, whisk together eggs, egg whites, vanilla, milk and cinnamon. Preheat a large nonstick skillet or griddle and spray with nonstick cooking spray on medium heat. Dunk each slice of bread into the egg mixture and saturate on both sides, about 1 minute per side. Then place in skillet. Repeat this with the other slices. Cook on one side until lightly brown, then turn over and cook until the other side is browned, about 2 minutes per side. Serve with pure maple syrup and optional fresh berries (or thawed frozen berries).

Pour any leftover egg mixture over the bread while cooking and use any day-old bread, even the ends!

Per serving (90 grams): 136 calories, 3.5 grams fat, 162 milligrams sodium, 21.6 grams carbohydrates, 4.2 grams dietary fiber, 8.8 grams protein.

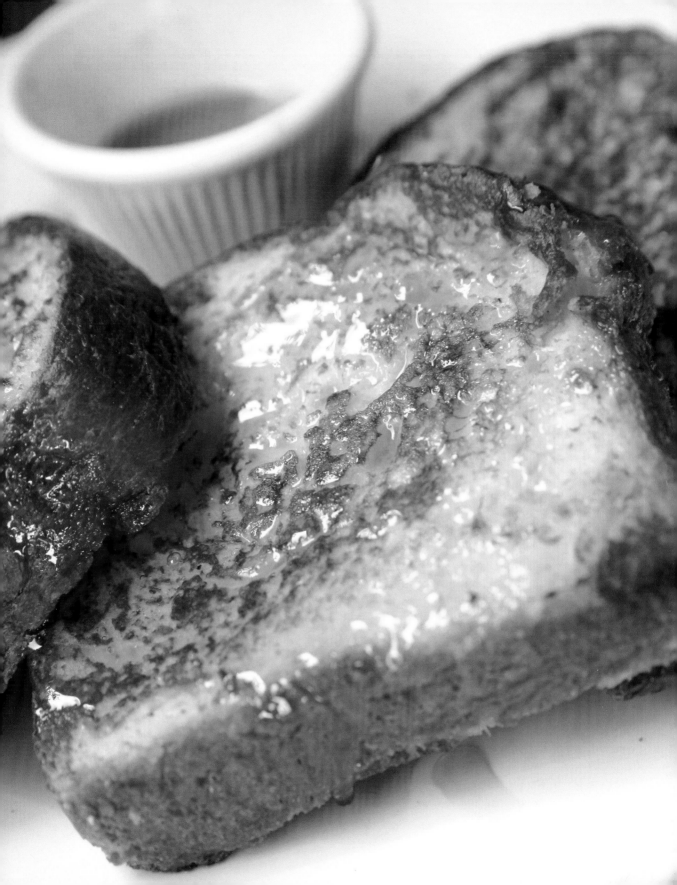

PLUM QUICK BREAD

Serves 10

(Requires soaking overnight)
1 cup all-purpose, unbleached flour
½ teaspoon baking powder
1 teaspoon baking soda
½ teaspoon ground cinnamon
½ teaspoons salt
½ cup organic sugar
2 cups whole-wheat flour
1 egg, slightly beaten
1 cup low-fat buttermilk
1 cup pitted prunes, chopped and soaked
  overnight in ½ cup prune juice
Nonstick cooking spray, olive oil

Preheat oven to 350 degrees Fahrenheit.

In a large bowl combine all-purpose flour, baking powder, baking soda, cinnamon, salt and sugar, and whisk to aerate. Then add whole-wheat flour and whisk again to combine thoroughly.

In a separate medium bowl, combine egg, buttermilk and prunes with prune juice. Pour wet ingredients into flour mixture and stir just enough to moisten the dry ingredients. Do not overmix.

Evenly spread the thick batter into a nonstick loaf pan (about 9-inch by 5-inch) lightly sprayed with nonstick cooking spray. Bake for an hour or until a knife comes out clean when inserted in the middle. Allow to cool; then remove from loaf pan, slice and serve.

This quick bread is also satisfying with afternoon tea.

Per serving (101 grams): 218 calories, 1 gram fat, 275 milligrams sodium, 49 grams carbohydrates, 2.6 grams dietary fiber, 4.8 grams protein.

BANANA DATE CHIA SEED MUFFINS

Serves 12

½ cup pitted dates
½ cup water
1½ cup mashed bananas (about 3 large
  bananas)
⅓ cup plain nonfat yogurt
3 tablespoons natural applesauce
1 teaspoon vanilla extract
1 egg plus 2 egg whites, lightly beaten
1 cup whole-wheat flour
¾ cup all-purpose, unbleached flour
¼ cup ground flaxseed
½ cup poppy seeds, divided in half
½ cup chia seeds, divided in half
½ teaspoon ground cinnamon
2 teaspoons baking powder
½ teaspoon salt
Nonstick cooking spray, olive oil

Preheat oven to 350 degrees Fahrenheit.

In a food processor or blender, puree dates with ½ cup water until smooth. To date puree, add bananas, yogurt, applesauce, vanilla, egg and egg whites. Blend and set mixture aside. In a separate large bowl, whisk the flours, flaxseed, ¼ cup poppy seeds, ¼ cup chia seeds, cinnamon, baking powder and salt. Fold the wet ingredients into the dry until just incorporated. Do not overmix! Evenly pour the mixture into 12 nonstick muffin tins lightly sprayed with nonstick cooking spray. Sprinkle with remaining ¼ cup chia and ¼ cup poppy seeds. Bake for 20 to 30 minutes or until golden brown and a knife inserted in the middle comes out clean. Allow to cool, then serve.

These muffins do not have added sugar, so don't expect a pastry-like sweetness. The dates, banana and applesauce add natural sweetness and a satisfying, moist texture.

Per muffin (89 grams): 181 calories, 5.8 grams fat, 121 milligrams sodium, 28.4 grams carbohydrates, 5.2 grams dietary fiber, 6.6 grams protein.

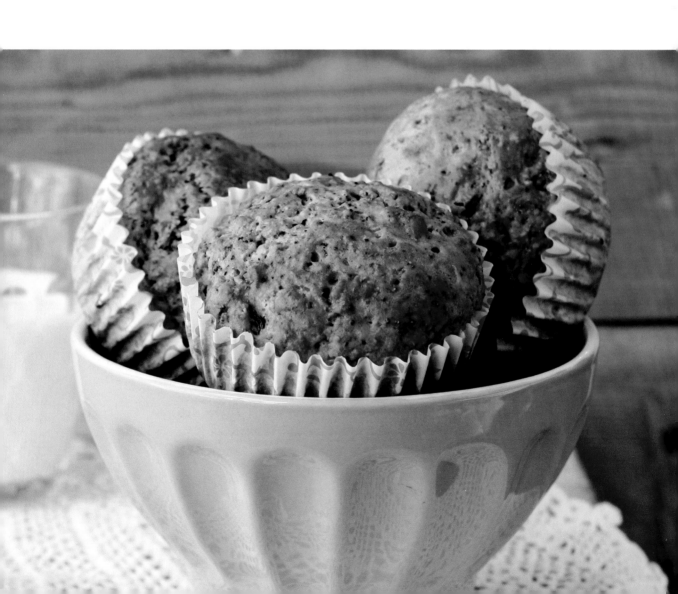

FARMER CHEESE, OLIVE AND RED PEPPER SPREAD

Serves 4

8 tablespoons of Farmer cheese
8 olives, preferably Kalamata, pitted, drained and chopped
1 whole roasted red pepper, drained and chopped
Freshly ground black pepper to taste

In a medium bowl, mix Farmer cheese, olives and red pepper; season with pepper and set aside.

Evenly divide the spread and serve with toasted sprouted-grain bread.

Prepare this a day or two ahead of time so flavors have time to blend.

Sprouted-grain bread has a low glycemic index and is high in protein and minerals compared to other breads. Glycemic index is a system that ranks foods on a scale from one to 100 based on their effect on blood-sugar levels. Sprouted-grain, whole-grain, multi-grain and sourdough breads are all good choices for people with diabetes, as part of a healthy diet.

Per serving without bread (57 grams): 65 calories, 3.5 grams fat, 240 milligrams sodium, 1.7 grams carbohydrates, 0.5 grams dietary fiber, 5.2 grams protein.

LOW-CARB/HIGH-PROTEIN BREAKFAST PANCAKES

Serves 4

2 eggs plus 2 egg whites, lightly beaten
¼ cup ground golden flaxseed
½ cup part-skim ricotta cheese
¾ teaspoon baking powder
¼ teaspoon salt
1 teaspoon stevia powder
Nonstick cooking spray, olive oil

In a large bowl, combine all ingredients and stir well. If the batter is too thick, add water. If it's too loose, add more ground flaxseed.

Heat a large nonstick skillet on medium-high heat and spray with cooking spray.

Pour one-quarter of the batter into skillet to make a pancake. Cook until golden on both sides, about 2 minutes per side. Repeat to make three more pancakes. Serve with sliced seasonal fruit and pure maple syrup or with part-skim ricotta cheese and jam.

For passed hors d'oeuvres or to make bite-size pancakes, divide the batter into eight servings and cook as instructed.

Per pancake (79 grams): 113 calories, 6.9 grams fat, 245 milligrams sodium, 4.3 grams carbohydrates, 2 grams dietary fiber, 9.6 grams protein.

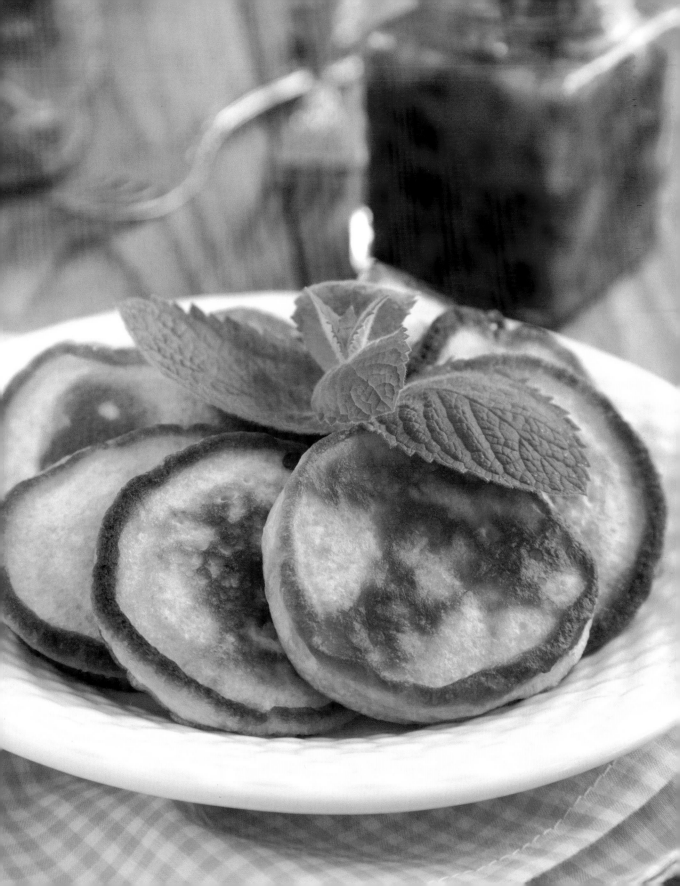

TOMATO BRUSCHETTA AND RICOTTA SPREAD

Serves 4

1 teaspoon extra-virgin olive oil
2 ripe plum tomatoes (or 2 small tomatoes
    on the vine), chopped
¼ cup fresh basil, chopped
⅛ teaspoon sea salt
Freshly ground black pepper, to taste
4 tablespoons part-skim or lite ricotta
    cheese, divided

In a medium bowl, combine oil, tomatoes, basil, salt and pepper. Evenly divide and serve on toasted olive or sourdough bread. Finish with a dollop (1 tablespoon each) of ricotta cheese and serve.

When buying part-skim or lite ricotta cheese, avoid brands made with gums like carrageenan. Ingredients should be: part skim milk, vinegar and salt. Nothing else!

Tomato bruschetta can be served over baked fish or with roasted chicken. It tastes great as a complement to any meal or as the main attraction at breakfast.

Per serving without bread (80 grams): 46 calories, 2.5 grams fat, 86 milligrams sodium, 4 grams carbohydrates, 0.7 grams dietary fiber, 2.6 grams protein.

SMOKED SALMON SPREAD

Serves 4

1 cup nonfat plain Greek yogurt
2 ounces organic or wild smoked salmon
    (no added nitrites), finely chopped
1 teaspoon dried dill weed or
    1 tablespoon fresh dill weed
½ cup fresh tomatoes, chopped (optional,
    for garnish)

In a medium bowl, combine ingredients and divide evenly. Serve with multi-grain toast. Garnish with optional chopped tomatoes and serve.

For a brunch buffet, serve a dollop of this smoked salmon spread on top of cucumber slices.

When serving bread, mix varieties of whole-grain, multi-grain, sprouted-grain, sourdough and other favorites.

Per serving without bread and without tomatoes (71 grams): 52 calories, 0.6 grams fat, 308 milligrams sodium, 2.6 grams carbohydrates, 1 gram dietary fiber, 8.6 grams protein.

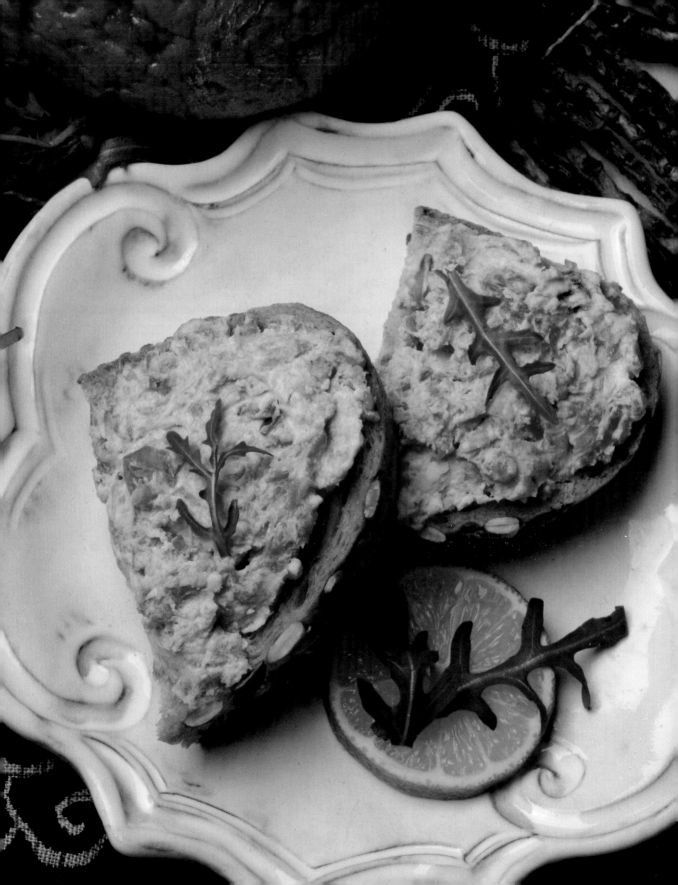

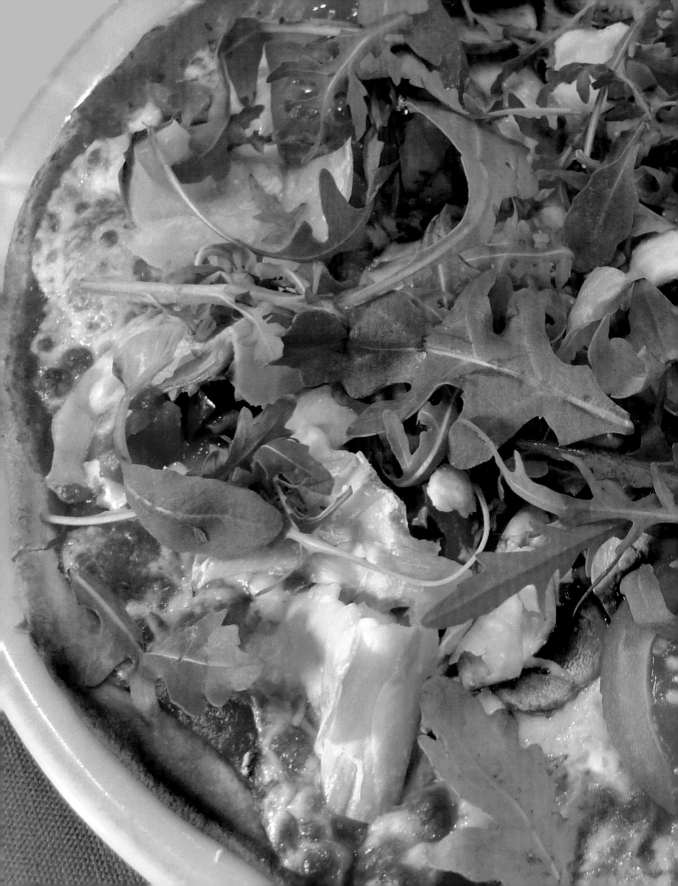

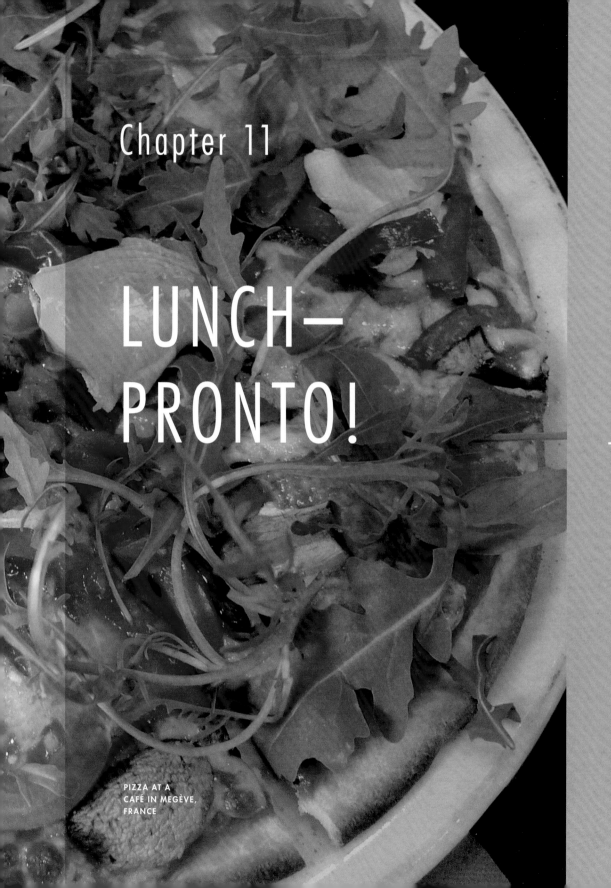

Chapter 11

LUNCH—PRONTO!

PIZZA AT A
CAFÉ IN MEGÈVE,
FRANCE

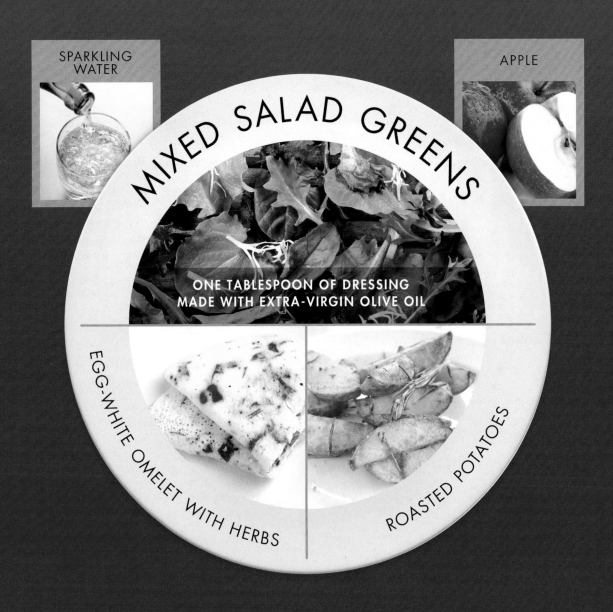

SPARKLING WATER

APPLE

MIXED SALAD GREENS

ONE TABLESPOON OF DRESSING
MADE WITH EXTRA-VIRGIN OLIVE OIL

EGG-WHITE OMELET WITH HERBS

ROASTED POTATOES

SUPER-HEALTHY LUNCH PLATE GUIDE

Knowing that Americans enjoy smaller lunches and larger dinners, these lunch recipes are sure to satisfy both your taste buds and appetite! If you're still hungry, add a broth-based soup or a lightly dressed salad. And if you're super-active, increase your serving size. On those occasions when lunch is the heavier meal, plan to lighten up at dinner. You can reverse the recipes for lunch and dinner, so mix, match and modify according to your needs!

Since greens are a nutritional powerhouse packed with vitamins, minerals, fiber and antioxidants, lunch is a perfect time to enjoy them. During summer, serve lunch over a heap of baby salad greens or arugula. During winter, complement a hearty lunch with steamed greens like kale, collards or Swiss chard. Baby spinach is a year-round staple: It can be enjoyed both raw and wilted (slightly cooked). It's easy to microwave washed greens: One to two minutes in a microwave-safe dish is all it takes.

While most Europeans don't eat eggs for breakfast, they enjoy omelets for a quick and healthy lunch. One large egg averages 70 calories and is an excellent and economical source of protein, vitamins and minerals. The yolk contains the fat-soluble vitamins (A, D and E) and most of the folic acid. Dietary choline, part of the vitamin B-complex, is also found in the yolk and is known to reduce inflammation and produce "happiness hormones" like serotonin, dopamine and norepinephrine. Like anything else, don't overdo it: Limit yourself to four whole eggs per week. If you're cutting back on cholesterol, substitute two egg whites for one whole egg. One large egg white contains 17 calories and about 60 percent of the protein (3.6 grams). Egg whites are naturally fat-free, cholesterol-free and provide selenium, potassium and magnesium. Choose organic, pasture-raised eggs or buy them from a local farm.

Enjoy the opportunity to expand your repertoire of recipes, as there are endless ways to create delicious omelets, pizzas, salads, soups and open-faced sandwiches. Pay attention to presentation: The more eye-appealing the food, the better it tastes.

187

LUNCH RECIPES

ROASTED TURKEY WITH SPICY CRANBERRY SAUCE ON TOAST

Serves 4

½ cup whole cranberry sauce (homemade or canned)
1 tablespoon walnuts, chopped
2 teaspoons Dijon mustard
1 teaspoon prepared white horseradish
4 ounces cooked, thinly sliced, roasted turkey breast, natural
4 romaine lettuce leaves
4 slices of sourdough, toasted
2 tablespoons flat-leaf parsley, chopped (garnish)

In a medium bowl, thoroughly combine cranberry sauce, walnuts, mustard and horseradish.

Place a lettuce leaf on each slice of toast. Equally divide and spread the cranberry mixture on the lettuce, then top each with 1 ounce of turkey. Garnish with parsley and serve.

Sourdough may have added health benefits. The fermentation and long rising time appears to break down starches, proteins, gluten and phytates, making the bread easier to digest. Sourdough has a lower glycemic index (68) compared to other breads (100). Some individuals with gluten intolerance may tolerate sourdough.

Per serving (119 grams): 200 calories, 2.3 grams fat, 300 milligrams sodium, 34.7 grams carbohydrates, 3.8 grams dietary fiber, 10.7 grams protein.

SHRIMP WITH CREAMY AVOCADO ON THIN RYE

Serves 4

4 tablespoons nonfat plain Greek yogurt
2 teaspoons fresh lime juice
⅛ teaspoon ground pink peppercorns
¼ avocado, chopped
8 large cooked shrimp (about 10 ounces), preservative-free
2 tablespoons flat-leaf parsley, chopped
4 slices thinly sliced rye bread, toasted

Combine yogurt, lime juice, ground peppercorns, and avocado; evenly spread on bread. Top with shrimp and then parsley. Serve open-faced.

Practice serving and eating open-faced sandwiches more often. You may find that you only need one slice of bread to feel satisfied.

Avocado by itself is a satisfying spread. One-fifth of a medium avocado (or 1 ounce) contains 50 calories, 4.5 grams fat (mostly monounsaturated), 3 grams carbohydrate, 2 grams dietary fiber and nearly 20 vitamins and minerals, including vitamin E.

Use avocado instead of mayo on any sandwich. Try it sprinkled with ground Espelette pepper.

Per serving (121 grams): 154 calories, 2.9 grams fat, 280 milligrams sodium, 15.2 grams carbohydrates, 1.9 grams dietary fiber, 16.6 grams protein.

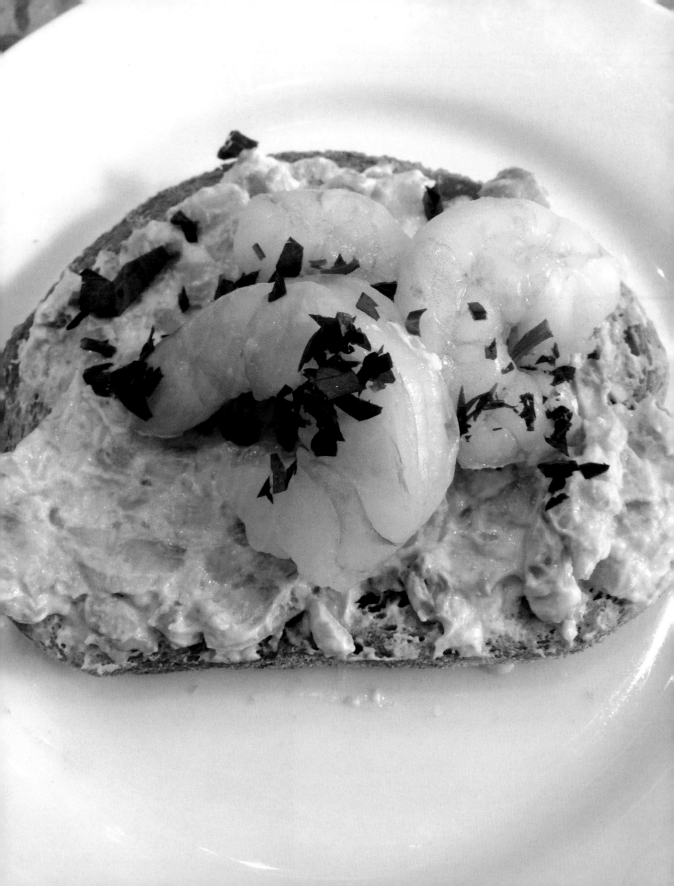

LENTILS, ROASTED BEETS AND TABOULEH OVER ARUGULA

Serves 4

For the Lentils:
1 cup green, red, yellow or brown lentils, rinsed
1½ cups water

Vinaigrette Dressing for Lentils
1 tablespoon extra-virgin olive oil
2 tablespoons red wine vinegar
2 teaspoons lime juice
¼ medium red onion, chopped
½ cup fresh flat-leaf parsley, chopped
4 cups arugula, chopped
Freshly ground sea salt to taste (optional)
Freshly ground black pepper to taste
   (optional)

In a medium pot, bring 1½ cups water to a boil. Add the lentils and turn the heat down to a simmer, stirring occasionally until lentils are tender. Drain and set aside. Cooking time will vary from 20 to 40 minutes, based on the variety of lentil. (Red lentils cook the quickest.) In a large bowl, whisk the olive oil, vinegar, lime juice, onion and parsley. Add the lentils to this vinaigrette and toss to combine. Season with salt and pepper if desired; serve over arugula.

Per serving for lentils and dressing only (94 grams): 193 calories, 4.7 grams fat, 15 milligrams sodium, 29 grams carbohydrates, 7.7 grams dietary fiber, 10.8 grams protein.

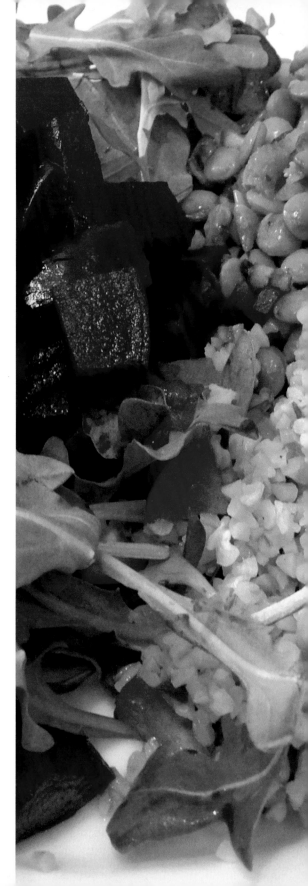

For the Roasted Beets:

2 pounds beets (about 6 medium beets)

3 tablespoons honey

Preheat oven to 375 degrees Fahrenheit.

Carefully scrub the beets and cut off the leaves and the long root tip. Save the beet greens and steam them separately later. Tightly wrap beets in foil and place in oven for 40 to 50 minutes or until the beets are tender and the skin is loose. Remove from oven and carefully open the foil to allow the steam to escape.

Allow the beets to cool enough so that you can handle them. Peel off the outer layer. It should slip off easily. If not then perhaps the beets need a bit more cooking. Cut the peeled beets into sixths or eighths—depending on the size of your beets. Drizzle with honey and serve.

Per serving for beets only (243 grams): 148 calories, 0 grams fat, 175 milligrams sodium, 35.6 grams carbohydrates, 4.6 grams dietary fiber, 3.9 grams protein.

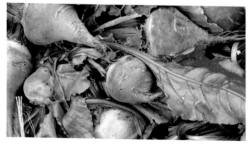

FRESH BEETS AT A FARMERS MARKET IN FRANCE

For the Tabouleh:

¾ cup uncooked bulgur

¾ cup water, boiled

4 cups tomatoes, diced

⅔ cup flat-leaf parsley, finely chopped

½ cup scallions, finely diced

2 lemons, juice only

1 tablespoon red wine vinegar

2 tablespoons extra-virgin olive oil

Freshly ground sea salt to taste (optional)

Freshly ground black pepper to taste (optional)

Place bulgur in a large bowl and cover with ¾ cup boiling water. Stir, then cover with a towel and allow to soak for an hour. In a separate medium bowl, combine tomatoes, parsley, scallions, lemon juice, vinegar and olive oil. Pour this mixture over the tabouleh and mix well. Season with optional salt and pepper, and serve.

Per serving for tabouleh only (244 grams): 195 calories, 7.8 grams fat, 21 milligrams sodium, 30.4 grams carbohydrates, 8.3 grams dietary fiber, 5.6 grams protein.

To Assemble:

Evenly divide the lentils, beets and tabouleh and arrange on four plates.

Cook these dishes ahead of time and use them individually as side dishes for dinner or over a heap of salad greens for a light lunch.

191

POACHED EGGS *PIPÉRADE*

Serves 2

2 teaspoons extra-virgin olive oil
1 white onion, coarsely chopped, (about
    1¼ cups)
1 cup mix of red, yellow and orange bell
    peppers, coarsely chopped
1 garlic clove, minced
3 large plum tomatoes, seeded and
    coarsely chopped
4 large eggs
¼ cup crumbled feta cheese (or 1 ounce)
Ground Espelette pepper or hot paprika
    to taste

Heat oil in a large skillet on medium heat. Add onion, peppers and garlic and sauté until soft, about 5 minutes. Add tomatoes and sauté until soft, about 3 minutes. Spread mixture evenly in skillet. Break eggs over vegetable mixture, spacing evenly. Cover skillet and reduce heat to low. Cook for about 5 minutes; yolk will still be soft.

Use a wide spatula and transfer 2 eggs with veggies underneath to each plate. Sprinkle with feta cheese and spoon remaining veggies around egg and season with pepper (or hot paprika). Serve with crusty whole-grain or sourdough bread.

Since the 16th century, Espelette pepper known in French as "piment d'Espelette," has been grown exclusively in Espelette, a small village in the French Basque Country. It has

a bold, warm and slightly smoky flavor. Hot paprika may be used as a substitution.

Pipérade is a famous dish also from the Basque region of France and is a sautéed mixture of onions, peppers and tomatoes, often paired with eggs—as in this recipe. Red, yellow and orange peppers provide a good dose of antioxidants including vitamin C.

Alternatively, prepare this recipe without the feta cheese.

Per serving with feta cheese (499 grams): 334 calories, 19.3 grams fat, 387 milligrams sodium, 23.7 grams carbohydrates, 5.1 grams dietary fiber, 19.6 grams protein.

ROASTED RATATOUILLE

Serves 4

1 small eggplant, cut into 1-inch pieces
1 small zucchini or yellow summer squash,
    cut into ¾-inch-thick slices
1 red bell pepper, cut into strips
½ small red onion, cut into ½-inch-thick
    wedges
1 tablespoon extra-virgin olive oil
½ teaspoon herbes de Provence or thyme,
    dried
¼ teaspoon freshly ground sea salt
⅛ teaspoon freshly ground black pepper
2 plum tomatoes, each cut lengthwise into
    6 wedges
2 tablespoons balsamic vinegar

Fresh thyme sprigs for garnish (optional)
Nonstick cooking spray, olive oil

Preheat oven to 400 degrees Fahrenheit.

Coat a large shallow roasting pan with nonstick cooking spray. (For a really quick clean-up, first line the pan with foil, then spray the foil with the cooking spray.) Add eggplant, zucchini, peppers and red onion to prepared pan. Drizzle with olive oil and sprinkle with herbes de Provence, salt and black pepper. Toss to coat.

Roast vegetables for 30 minutes, tossing once. Add plum tomatoes to roasting pan. Roast for another 15 to 20 minutes or until vegetables are tender. Sprinkle with balsamic vinegar before serving. Garnish with thyme sprigs. Serve with brown rice or crusty bread.

Ratatouille is a delicious vegetable side dish to be served with any meal. Try it for breakfast on a slice of toast, topped with olive tapenade.

Per serving (166 grams): 68 calories, 3.8 grams fat, 162 milligrams sodium, 7.9 grams carbohydrates, 2.1 grams dietary fiber, 1.8 grams protein.

TOMATO, MOZZARELLA AND SWISS CHARD FRITTATA

Serves 4

1 tablespoon extra-virgin olive oil
½ cup shallots, chopped
4 ounces Swiss chard, chopped

4 whole eggs plus 4 egg whites, lightly beaten
8 cherry or grape tomatoes, halved
2 ounces part-skim mozzarella, shredded or chopped
2 tablespoons fresh basil, chopped
Freshly ground black pepper to taste (optional)

Preheat the oven to 425 degrees Fahrenheit.

Heat the oil in a large ovenproof skillet (or cast iron skillet) over medium heat. Add the shallots and cook for 5 minutes, stirring often, until softened.

Add the chard and cook until just wilted, 2 to 3 minutes. Pour the eggs over the Swiss chard.

Scatter the tomatoes, mozzarella and basil on top. They should sink slightly.

Lower the heat slightly and cook until mostly set, about 5 minutes.

Transfer to the oven and bake for 5 to 10 minutes (ovens vary—mine took 9 minutes) until fully set and cooked through.

Remove from the oven and allow to cool slightly.

Cut into slices and serve with a green salad and a slice of crusty bread. (Tastes delicious the next day too.)

Per serving (391 grams): 209 calories, 10.7 grams fat, 279 milligrams sodium, 15 grams carbohydrates, 3.5 grams dietary fiber, 15.8 grams protein.

193

MUSHROOM AND SALMON QUICHE (CRUSTLESS)

Serves 8

2 large eggs plus 2 egg whites
1 cup nonfat plain Greek yogurt
1 tablespoon whole-wheat flour
½ teaspoon baking soda
Freshly ground black pepper to taste
Freshly ground sea salt to taste (optional)
1 cup (your favorite) mushrooms, chopped
4 ounces cooked salmon, shredded
1 cup reduced-fat cheddar cheese, grated
2 tablespoons flat-leaf parsley, chopped
Nonstick cooking spray, olive oil

Preheat oven to 450 degrees Fahrenheit.

In a blender, combine eggs, egg whites and yogurt. Add flour, baking soda, pepper and optional salt. Blend again. Pour mixture into a large bowl. Add mushrooms and salmon to the mixture and stir. Spray a 9-inch round baking dish (or pie plate) with cooking spray. Pour mixture into the baking dish.

Layer cheese on top. Garnish with parsley. Bake for 15 minutes, then reduce heat to 350 degrees Fahrenheit and bake 15 to 20 minutes more. Tent the top if the cheese browns quickly. Allow quiche to set for 5 minutes before serving.

Alternatively, use smoked salmon instead of cooked salmon. Always check the ingredient label to make sure the salmon is preservative-free and naturally smoked. Opt for organically farmed or wild varieties.

Per serving (88 grams): 110 calories, 5.9 grams fat, 234 milligrams sodium, 3.8 grams carbohydrates, 0.7 grams dietary fiber, 11.3 grams protein.

CLASSIC MINESTRONE SOUP

Serves 6

1 tablespoon extra-virgin olive oil
1 medium onion, diced
2 carrots, diced
1½ cups Savoy or Napa cabbage, chopped
½ pound green beans, cleaned, ends removed and cut in thirds
14 ounces diced tomatoes
15 ounces kidney or pinto beans (canned or cooked), drained and rinsed
1 large potato, peeled and diced
1 cup peas, fresh or frozen (if frozen, thaw)
2 cups strained tomatoes
2 cups vegetable broth, low-sodium
1 teaspoon oregano, dried (or 1 tablespoon fresh)
1 teaspoon basil, dried (or 1 tablespoon fresh)
1 bay leaf
½ teaspoon red pepper flakes
Freshly ground sea salt to taste (optional)

194

Heat oil in a large stockpot over medium heat and sauté onions for 2 minutes. Add carrots and cabbage and sauté 2 minutes. Stir in green beans and sauté 1 minute. Add diced tomatoes, kidney (or pinto) beans, potato, peas, strained tomatoes and broth and bring to a boil.

Lower heat, then add herbs and pepper; then simmer for 20 minutes. Remove bay leaf before serving.

For a complete-protein vegetarian meal, serve with freshly grated Parmesan cheese and hearty whole-grain bread. Be adventurous and add extra vegetables that may be lurking in your fridge. If you fancy garlic, add a clove while you're sautéing the onion.

Per serving (482 grams, about 2 cups): 220 calories, 3.2 grams fat, 312 milligrams sodium, 38.4 grams carbohydrates, 12.3 grams dietary fiber, 11.4 grams protein.

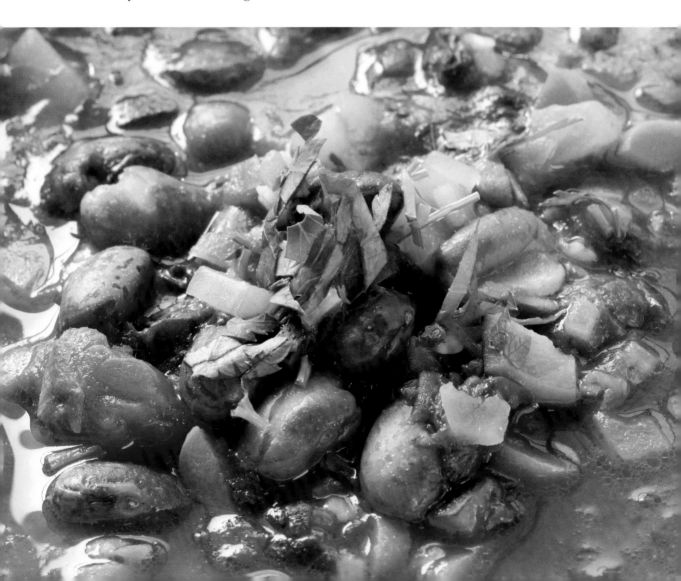

PORTABELLO MUSHROOM PIZZA

Serves 2

2 Portabello mushrooms, cleaned and
   stemmed (or 6 ounces)
2 teaspoons extra-virgin olive oil, divided
Freshly ground sea salt to taste (optional)
Freshly ground black pepper to taste
1 tomato, chopped and divided
½ teaspoon dried oregano
2 ounces fresh mozzarella cheese
2 tablespoons fresh basil

Preheat the oven to 400 degrees
Fahrenheit.

Heat 1 teaspoon of olive oil in a
medium-sized nonstick saucepan over
medium heat. Place the Portabello
mushrooms in the pan with the fleshy
part facing up and the cap facing
down. Drizzle mushrooms with
1 teaspoon of olive oil and season with
optional salt and pepper. Evenly top
the two mushrooms with the chopped
tomato and season with oregano.

Reduce the heat to medium-low
and place a lid over the saucepan.
Cook the mushrooms for 5 minutes or
until softened. Open lid and evenly
distribute cheese over the tomatoes.
Simmer with lid on for 3 more minutes
or until cheese is melted.

Garnish with fresh basil and serve
with focaccia bread.

Per serving without bread (152 grams): 155 calories,
10.6 grams fat, 156 milligrams sodium, 6.9 grams
carbohydrates, 1.9 grams dietary fiber, 9.9 grams protein.

MOSTLY EGG-WHITE OMELET WITH SPINACH AND SUN-DRIED TOMATO

Serves 2

1 egg plus 4 egg whites
1 ounce or 2 tablespoons fat-free milk
⅛ teaspoon ground white, Espelette or
   black pepper
2 tablespoons fresh basil, chopped
1 cup baby spinach, chopped
4 sun-dried tomatoes, rehydrated* and
   chopped (or ½ roasted red pepper,
   chopped)
Nonstick cooking spray, olive oil

In a medium bowl, whisk egg, egg
whites, milk and pepper until frothy.
In a separate medium bowl, combine
basil, spinach and sun-dried tomatoes
(or roasted red pepper).

Coat a large skillet with nonstick
spray and heat over medium heat for
1 minute. Pour egg mixture into pan
and cook until eggs begin to set. Spread
the filling over half the omelet, leaving
a ½-inch border. Lift up edge and,
when lightly browned on bottom, fold
in half. Cook 1 to 2 minutes more and
slide onto plate. Cut in half and serve
with crusty bread.

*To rehydrate sun-dried tomatoes,
place them in a microwave-safe
glass bowl and cover with water.
Microwave on high for 1 minute. Let
stand for 5 minutes. If they are still
tough, microwave again for 1 more

minute. When water is cooled, remove the sun-dried tomatoes and use in your recipe. Alternatively, substitute ½ roasted red pepper for sun-dried tomatoes.

There are so many ways to prepare egg-white omelets using an assortment of fresh herbs and vegetables. So experiment with what's on hand and Bon Appétit!

Per serving (124 grams): 83 calories, 2.5 grams fat, 240 milligrams sodium, 4.3 grams carbohydrates, 1 gram dietary fiber, 11.5 grams protein.

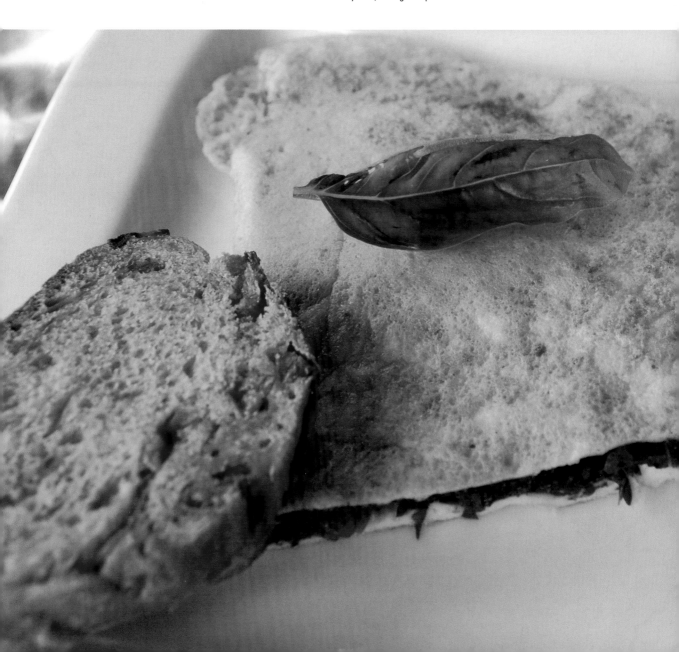

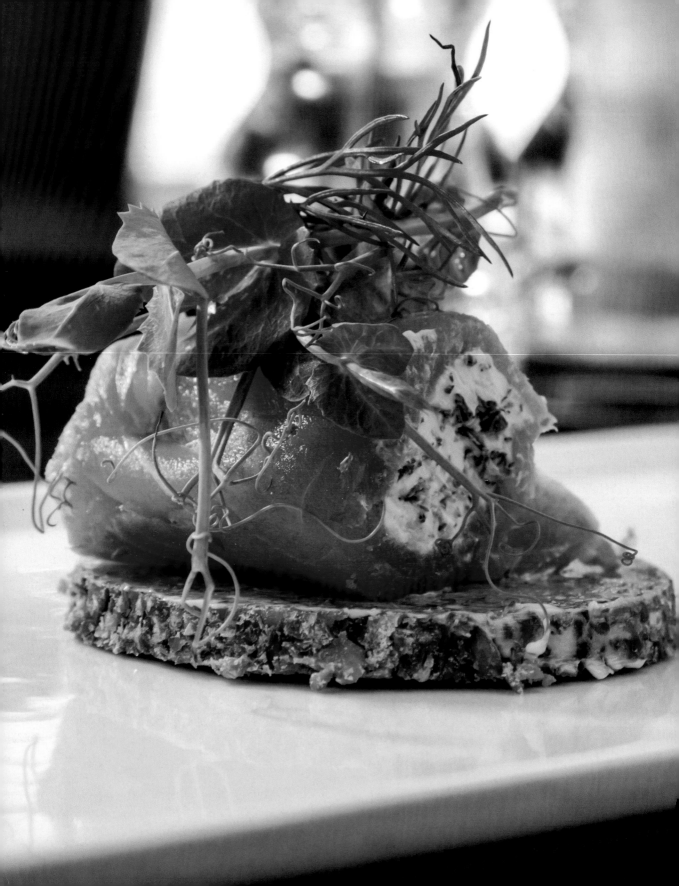

Chapter 12

SNACKS AND HORS D'OEUVRES

STRAINED NONFAT PLAIN GREEK
YOGURT AND HERBS WRAPPED
WITH WILD ALASKAN SMOKED
SALMON ON MULTI-GRAIN BREAD

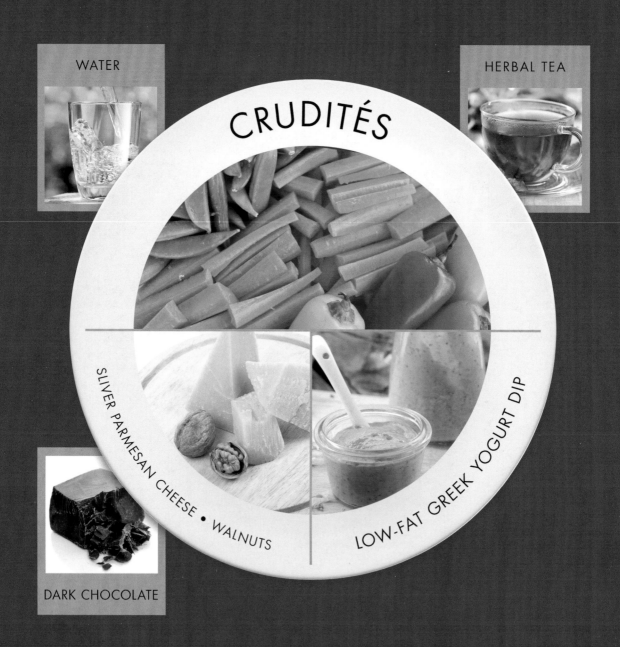

WATER

HERBAL TEA

CRUDITÉS

SLIVER PARMESAN CHEESE • WALNUTS

LOW-FAT GREEK YOGURT DIP

DARK CHOCOLATE

SUPER-HEALTHY SNACK PLATE GUIDE

S nacking is an American habit that can either improve your waistline by curbing your appetite or, if abused or incorrectly used, can expand your belly, leading to obesity.

By sticking to smaller portions at mealtimes, snacking can be useful in keeping blood sugars steady. On the other hand, eating larger portions at mealtimes and then racking up calories in between can become a dangerous habit.

Snacking should be thought of as a mini-meal, or an extension of your meals, and eaten only if you're hungry. A good habit is to cut your meal in half and eat the second half, if needed, as a snack two to three hours after breakfast, lunch or dinner. Remember to drink a glass of water before and in between meals to make sure you're staying hydrated. Often we think our body is telling us that we are hungry, when in reality, we are simply thirsty!

After breakfast, Europeans typically have a midmorning coffee or tea. Americans also enjoy a mid-morning coffee or tea, but feel inclined to add a muffin, brownie or donut. That's because the cashier will ask, "What else can I get you with your coffee?" In the U.S., we've become brainwashed to have a "treat" with coffee (or tea), rather than just enjoy a simple coffee (or tea) break.

This goes back to the food industry's practice of cross-merchandizing and selling more products. The corner coffee shop lines the counter with donuts, bagels, cookies and rolls, tempting you to buy more than just the coffee. And cereal companies invented cereal bars to compete with the "grab and go," midmorning, sugary snack category.

When it comes to snacks, choose foods that are as nutritious and wholesome as what you would eat at a meal. Avoid foods that are loaded with fat, sugar and salt, which become a dump of empty calories and salt into your body. What you want is a boost of energy, not a bloated belly making you feel tired and sluggish. If you're on the run, pack a banana and a nonfat yogurt. If you need some crunch, bring along twenty dry-roasted almonds and baby carrots. The bottom line is to snack mindfully and only if you need it!

201

SNACK RECIPES

"THIN" CHEESE CRÊPES

Serves 6

½ cup white whole-wheat flour
½ cup all-purpose flour
¼ teaspoon salt
2 large eggs plus 2 egg whites
½ cup fat-free milk or original almond milk
2 teaspoons extra-virgin olive oil
½ cup seltzer or sparkling water
6 ounces part-skim or lite ricotta cheese
6 teaspoons apricot fruit spread
   (100 percent fruit)
3 cups fresh seasonal fruit, diced

In a blender or food processor fitted with a stainless steel blade, combine whole-wheat flour, all-purpose flour, salt, eggs, egg whites, milk and oil until smooth, scraping the sides once or twice. Transfer to a bowl, cover and refrigerate for at least 30 minutes or overnight. Slowly whisk seltzer into the batter. Heat a large nonstick skillet sprayed with cooking spray over medium to high heat. Ladle ⅓ cup batter into the center of the pan. Immediately tilt and rotate the pan to spread the batter evenly over the bottom. Cook until the underside is lightly browned, about 30 seconds to 1 minute. Using a heatproof silicon or rubber spatula, lift the edge and then quickly grasp the crêpe with your fingers and flip. Cook until the second side is lightly browned, about

20 seconds. Slide onto a plate. Repeat with the remaining batter, spraying the pan as needed and stacking crêpes as you go. If the pan begins to smoke, reduce the heat to medium. As you prepare your filling, cover crêpes with a paper towel or keep warm in a 200-degree Fahrenheit oven.

To assemble, place a crêpe on a clean cutting board. Spread 2 tablespoons of ricotta and 1 teaspoon of jam in the center, leaving a 1-to 2-inch border. Fold in the sides to make a square shape, leaving a "window" in the center. Press down on the corners, as necessary, to help keep the crêpe folded. Serve with ½ cup of fresh fruit per crêpe.

White whole-wheat flour, made from a special variety of white-wheat, is light in color and flavor but has the same nutritional properties as regular whole-wheat flour. It is available at large supermarkets and natural-foods stores and online at bobsredmill.com or kingarthurflour.com. Store it in the freezer.

For an easier version of this recipe, buy natural crêpe batter or prepared (pre-made) crêpes in your food market. Prepared (imported from France) crêpes are often sold in the produce aisle.

Per serving (204 grams): 207 calories, 5.9 grams fat, 198 milligrams sodium, 29.2 grams carbohydrates, 1.3 grams dietary fiber, 10 grams protein.

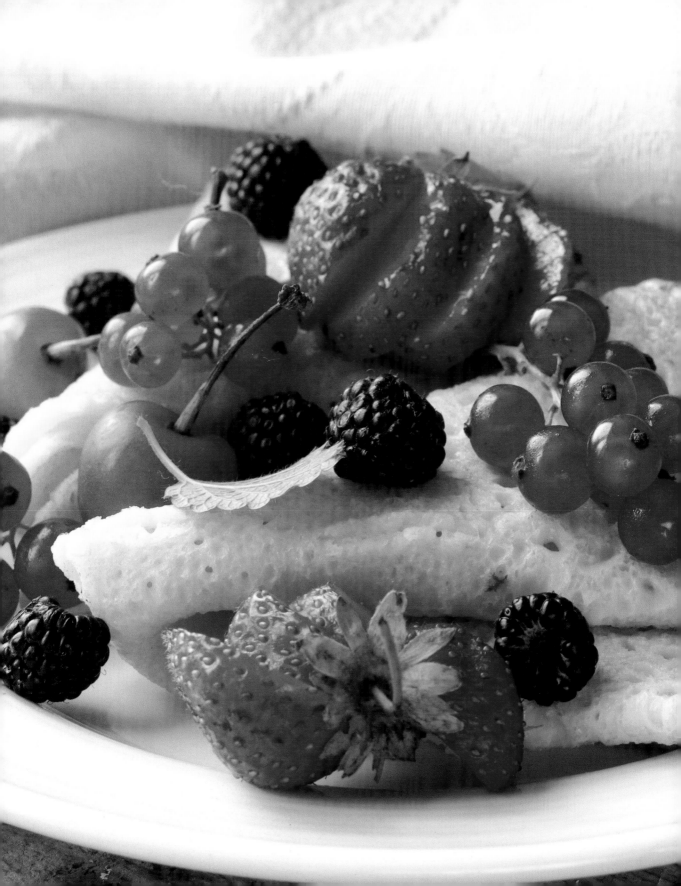

WALNUT HUMMUS (GARLIC-FREE AND OIL-FREE)

Serves 4

19 ounces chickpeas (garbanzo beans),
    rinsed and drained
¼ cup walnuts, chopped
3 tablespoons lemon juice
1 tablespoon water (more if needed)
Sea salt to taste (optional)
Freshly ground black pepper to taste
1 teaspoon cumin powder (optional)

In a blender or food processor fitted
with a stainless steel blade, combine
all ingredients and blend thoroughly.
Adjust consistency by adding water*
(or extra-virgin olive oil). Serve with
crudité—cut-up veggies.

*For fewer calories and less fat, use water
to adjust the consistency of the hummus.
There are 120 calories in 1 tablespoon of oil,
while water has zero calories.*

Per serving without added salt (158 grams): 197
calories, 5.9 grams fat, 37 milligrams sodium, 24.5 grams
carbohydrates, 6.2 grams dietary fiber, 9.9 grams protein.

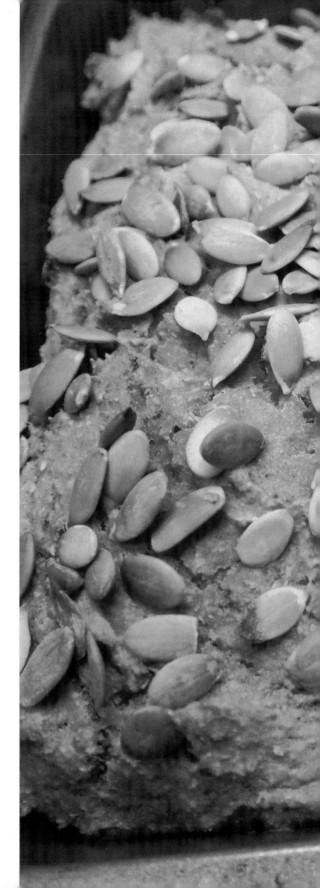

PUMPKIN SPICE QUICK BREAD

Serves 12

2 cups whole-wheat flour
½ cup organic sugar
½ teaspoon salt
1 teaspoon baking soda
1 teaspoon ground cinnamon
⅛ teaspoon ground cloves
⅛ teaspoon ground nutmeg
4 ounces applesauce
2 large eggs, lightly beaten
2 cups pumpkin puree (canned or fresh)
1 teaspoon vanilla
¼ cup pumpkin seeds (optional)
Nonstick cooking spray, olive oil

Preheat oven to 400 degrees Fahrenheit.

In a medium bowl, whisk together flour, sugar, salt, baking soda and spices. In a separate large bowl, whisk together applesauce, eggs, pumpkin puree and vanilla.

Slowly fold the wet ingredients into the dry; combine, but don't over mix. Spray a 9 x 5 x 3 inch loaf pan (or a shallow 8-inch baking pan) with cooking spray. Pour the batter into the prepared baking dish and sprinkle with optional pumpkin seeds.

Bake for 35 to 40 minutes, checking for doneness. Let cool for 15 minutes. Run a knife around the edges of the pan to loosen and un-mold. (This freezes well, so make an extra loaf.)

Alternatively, use this batter to make 12 muffins!

Per serving (92 grams): 155 calories, 2.5 grams fat, 215 milligrams sodium, 29.4 grams carbohydrates, 2 grams dietary fiber, 4.4 grams protein.

RICOTTA AND SMOKED SALMON WITH CUCUMBER

Serves 2

½ cup part-skim or lite ricotta cheese
1 ounce naturally smoked salmon (no added nitrites), finely chopped
1 teaspoon lemon juice
1 teaspoon dried dill weed (or 1 tablespoon fresh)
1 cucumber, ends removed and sliced lengthwise into 2-inch strips

Combine all ingredients (except cucumber) and serve with cucumber slices.

Serve also as a breakfast spread or as a filling for an omelet.

Per serving (230 grams): 129 calories, 5.9 grams fat, 144 milligrams sodium, 9 grams carbohydrate, 1 gram dietary fiber, 11 grams protein.

205

EGG-WHITE SOUFFLÉ IN TWO MINUTES

Serves 1

(Cook in a microwave)
2 egg whites or 2 ounces liquid egg whites
1 tablespoon part-skim or lite ricotta cheese
1 handful baby spinach, chopped
Pinch of sumac or sea salt (optional)
Freshly ground black pepper to taste (optional)

In a small bowl or ramekin—one that holds ½ to 1 cup liquid—using a fork, gently beat egg whites with ricotta. Fold in spinach. Cook in a microwave for 1 minute and 10 seconds. Season as desired and enjoy! Optional: Serve on a half of a whole-grain ciabatta roll.

This recipe takes only 2 minutes to prepare *and* cook, and requires only one *small* dish for mixing, cooking *and* eating! My son Ben Anapol is the creator!

If you don't have spinach on hand, try this with any vegetable or a combination of seasonal vegetables.

While traveling in Europe, I discovered sumac, a spice commonly used in Middle Eastern cuisine, which adds a lemony and slightly salty taste to salads, eggs and meats. Use sumac to replace salt in savory dishes.

Per serving without added salt (89 grams): 55 calories, 1.4 grams fat, 135 milligrams sodium, 1.6 grams carbohydrates, 9.2 grams protein.

CHOCOLATE TOFU BANANA MOUSSE

Serves 4

1 banana, broken into chunks
12 ounces firm tofu, silken preferred
¼ cup pure maple syrup
2 tablespoons blackstrap molasses (optional)
5 tablespoons unsweetened cocoa powder
3 tablespoons (or 1½ ounces) fat-free milk or original almond milk
¼ teaspoon ground cinnamon

In a blender, combine banana, tofu, maple syrup, optional molasses, cocoa powder, milk and cinnamon. Cover and puree until smooth. Pour into individual serving dishes or one shallow bowl and refrigerate for 1 hour before serving.

This was the "go-to" snack for my children when they were young. They loved it! Need I say more? And yes, it tastes as rich as velvety French mousse.

Per serving (164 grams): 135 calories, 2.5 grams fat, 19 milligrams sodium, 24 grams carbohydrates, 1 gram dietary fiber, 5.4 grams protein.

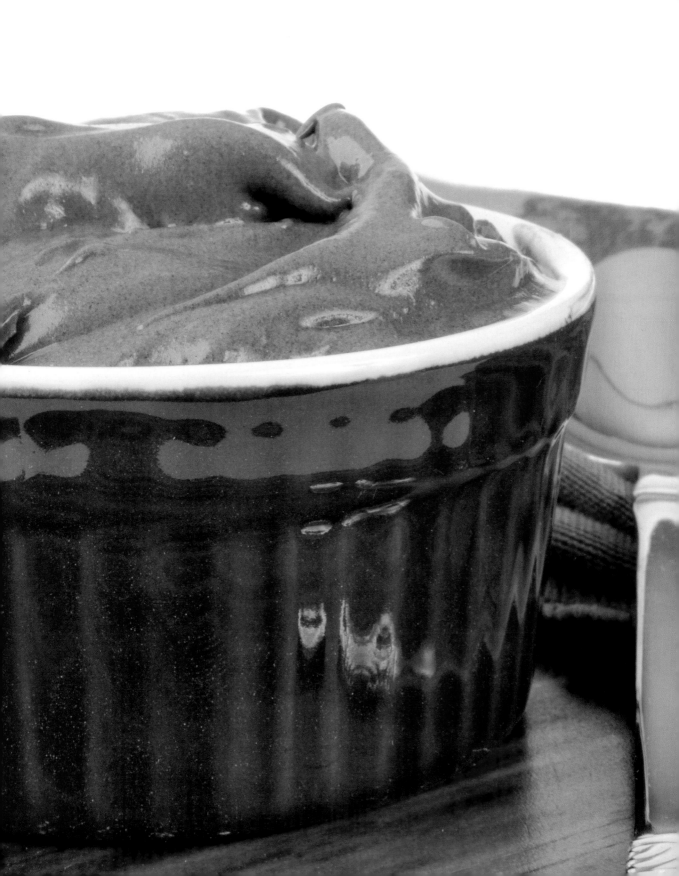

CREAMY SWEET POTATO CUSTARD

Serves 4

1¾ cups cooked sweet potato (canned or
    fresh*, from about 2 medium potatoes)
⅓ cup pure maple syrup
1 egg plus 2 egg whites, beaten
½ cup fat-free milk or original almond milk
1 teaspoon vanilla extract
2 tablespoons cornstarch
½ teaspoon ground cinnamon
¼ teaspoon ground nutmeg
¼ teaspoon ground ginger
Nonstick cooking spray, olive oil

Preheat oven to 350 degrees Fahrenheit.
    In a blender or food processor fitted
with a stainless steel blade, combine
all ingredients until smooth. Spray a
9-inch round glass baking dish with
nonstick cooking spray and pour sweet
potato mixture into baking dish. Bake
for 55 to 60 minutes or until set. Allow
to cool for 1 to 2 hours and serve at
room temperature or chilled.
    *If you are using fresh sweet
potatoes, peel and cut them in ½-inch
slices, then steam in a saucepan for
7 to 8 minutes. Cool and use them in
this recipe.

*Creamy sweet potatoes are satisfying
anytime of the day, and they are brimming
with vitamin A (beta carotene), vitamin C,
B-vitamins, potassium and fiber.*

Per serving (177 grams): 200 calories, 1.4 grams fat,
90 milligrams sodium, 41.6 grams carbohydrates, 3 grams
dietary fiber, 6 grams protein.

PETIT BEAN PATTIES

Serves 8

1 egg or 2 egg whites
⅓ cup cornmeal
¾ cup rolled oats
15 ounces black beans (canned or
    cooked) or lentils, rinsed and drained
½ red onion, chopped (or ½ cup)
½ teaspoon cumin powder
2 tablespoons ketchup
¼ teaspoon hot pepper oil
Nonstick cooking spray, olive oil

Combine all ingredients in a food
processor or blender fitted with a
stainless steel blade and pulse five
times. Wet hands and form into 8
small patties. Spray a large skillet with
cooking spray and heat on medium-
high heat. Place patties in skillet and
cook on each side for 2 to 3 minutes or
until done. Serve with your favorite
condiments.

*For veggie burger-style, make 4 larger
patties and serve for lunch or dinner. Both
beans and oats are excellent sources of
soluble fiber, the type of fiber that helps
reduce cholesterol and control blood sugar.*

Per serving made with egg whites (85 grams): 108 calories,
1.3 grams fat, 65 milligrams sodium, 18.7 grams
carbohydrates, 3.9 grams dietary fiber, 5.6 grams protein.

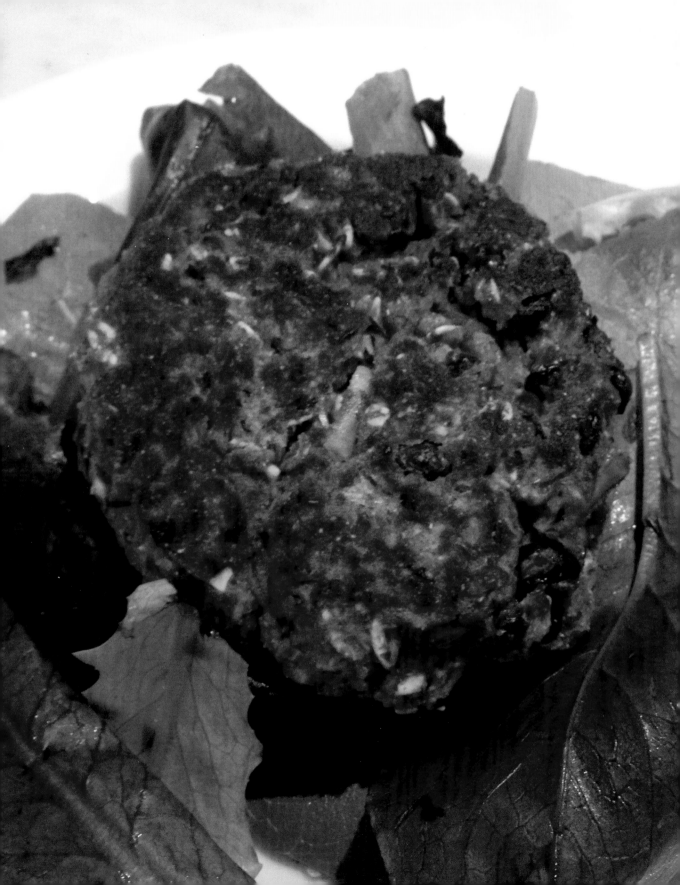

EGGLESS EGG SALAD LETTUCE ROLLS

Serves 3

1 cup or 8 ounces firm tofu, drained and
   excess water squeezed out
1 teaspoon apple cider vinegar
2 teaspoons Dijon mustard
1 teaspoon agave syrup or honey
½ teaspoon turmeric
¼ cup celery, finely chopped
2 tablespoons onion, finely chopped
1 tablespoon flat-leaf parsley, finely
   chopped
¼ teaspoon white pepper
3 romaine lettuce leaves, cleaned and
   dried

In a medium bowl, crumble tofu and
set aside. In a separate small bowl,
combine vinegar, mustard, agave or
honey and turmeric. Mix thoroughly
and pour over tofu. Add celery, onion,
parsley and pepper. Mix thoroughly
and refrigerate about 1 hour for flavors
to blend. Place one-third of the mixture
onto each of the lettuce leaves; roll and
serve.

*Also serve this eggless egg salad as an
open-faced sandwich for breakfast or on top
of a mixed green salad for lunch.*

Per serving (114 grams): 72 calories, 3.4 grams fat,
56 milligrams sodium, 5 grams carbohydrates, 1.7 grams
dietary fiber, 6.9 grams protein.

MANGO AND GREENS PICK-ME-UP SMOOTHIE

Serves 2

1 frozen banana
1 cup (packed) baby spinach
1 fresh mango, diced (about 1 cup)
1½ cups original almond milk

Combine all ingredients in a blender
and blend until smooth and serve.

*It's best to use frozen fruit rather than
add ice cubes to smoothies. The ice dilutes
the flavors, and the "coldness" reduces
the ability to taste the natural sweetness.
Our taste buds work better when food
and beverages are served close to room
temperature. That's why ice cream tastes
sweeter when it's melted.*

Per serving (365 grams): 168 calories, 2.6 grams fat,
127 milligrams sodium, 37.5 grams carbohydrates, 4.6 grams
dietary fiber, 2.4 grams protein.

210

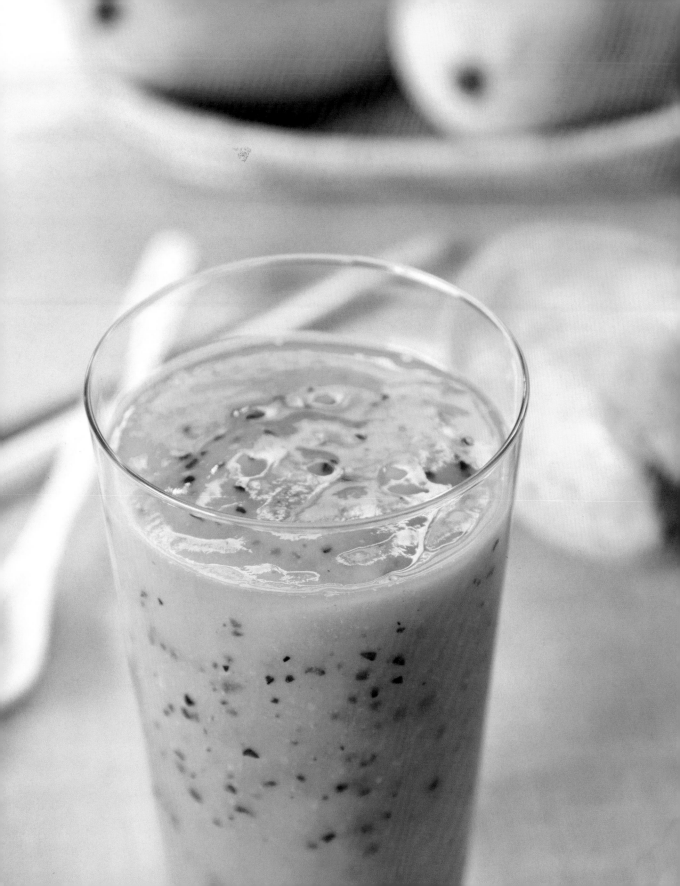

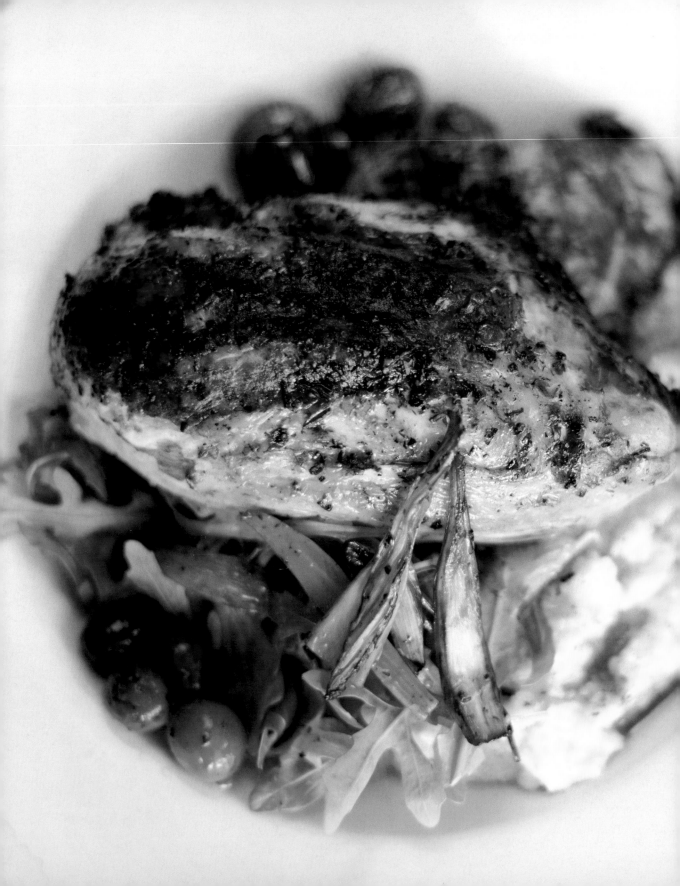

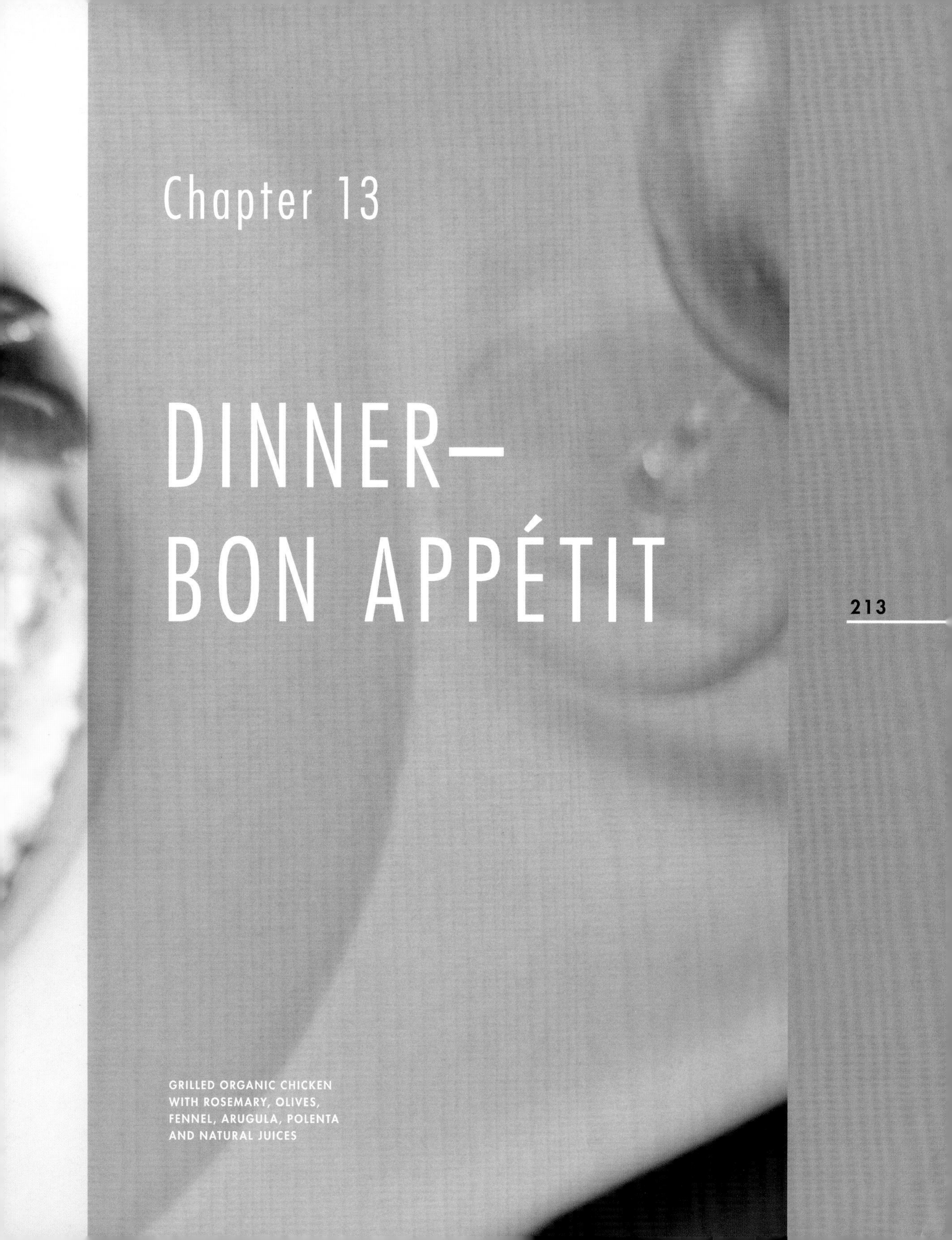

Chapter 13

DINNER— BON APPÉTIT

GRILLED ORGANIC CHICKEN
WITH ROSEMARY, OLIVES,
FENNEL, ARUGULA, POLENTA
AND NATURAL JUICES

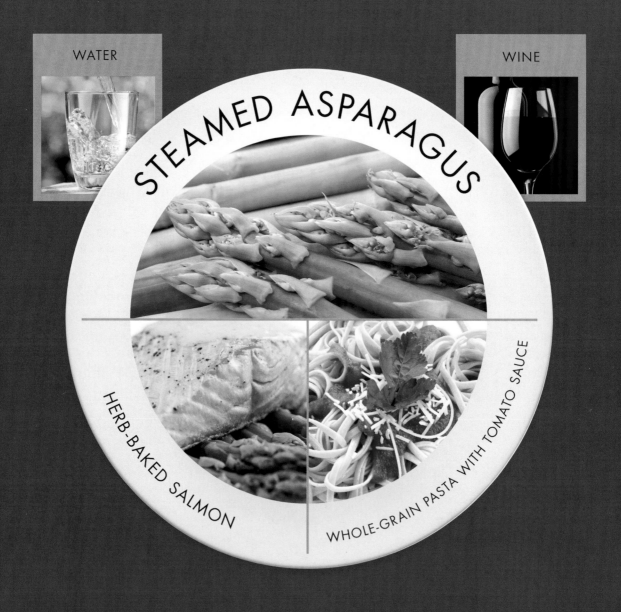

WATER

WINE

STEAMED ASPARAGUS

HERB-BAKED SALMON

WHOLE-GRAIN PASTA WITH TOMATO SAUCE

SUPER-HEALTHY DINNER PLATE GUIDE

T he calming ritual of a family dinner, as commonly practiced in Europe, can dramatically enhance your health and well-being. The dinner table is not only the place where traditions are passed down from one generation to the next, it's also the environment where a sense of security develops within a strong family framework.

In fact, those who share dinnertime are less likely to have eating disorders, more likely to eat healthy foods and less likely to be overweight. That's because at the family dinner table, you can control exactly what and how much you're going to eat.

When Europeans eat a large lunch out, they generally have a small dinner at home. They tend to be conscious of how much and which types of food they have eaten during the day. Then the evening meal is planned accordingly. For example, if meat, poultry or fish were had for lunch, then dinner might be pasta served with a salad or other appetizer. In contrast, we Americans don't often think about how much or what we've eaten for long-term planning purposes. For us, food represents the immediate gratification of whatever urge—burgers, candy, muffins—we might have at any given moment. Instead we need to plan our day with the right balance of choices to delight the palate and nourish the body.

Now, it's time to put on your chef's hat and decide what to have for dinner. First, consider what you ate for lunch. Then, start preparing a simple yet enticing dinner that will bring your family and friends back to the table again and again. The components of a successful dinner include delicious food, engaging conversation and a relaxing atmosphere.

DINNER RECIPES

CHICKEN CUTLETS WITH TOMATOES AND ONIONS

Serves 4

1 pound small chicken cutlets, about 8
⅛ teaspoon sea salt
Freshly ground black pepper to taste
1 tablespoon extra-virgin olive oil, divided
    into 3 teaspoons
1 onion, chopped (or 1 cup)
1½ pints cherry tomatoes, cut in half
¾ cup dry white wine
2 tablespoons fresh tarragon, chopped
2 tablespoons fresh basil, chopped

Lightly season the chicken with salt and pepper. Heat 1 teaspoon of oil in a large nonstick skillet on medium to high heat. If needed, work in batches and cook cutlets 2 to 3 minutes per side. Add another teaspoon of olive oil if needed. Transfer cooked cutlets to a plate dressed with baby arugula.

Add the final teaspoon of olive oil to the skillet and sauté onions for 5 minutes. Add tomatoes and cook 2 to 3 minutes. Add wine and turn heat down to a simmer. Cook for 2 to 3 minutes until liquid is reduced by half. Stir in tarragon and basil. Add the tomato-onion mixture to the chicken cutlets—on top or next to the cutlets—and serve.

216

This is a light dish that goes well with steamed green beans and any delicate grain like couscous or angel hair pasta.

Per serving (303 grams): 220 calories, 5.3 grams fat, 140 milligrams sodium, 8.5 grams carbohydrates, 2 grams dietary fiber, 27.6 grams protein.

QUINOA RISOTTO

Serves 6

2 teaspoons extra-virgin olive oil
1 onion, finely chopped (about 1 cup)
1 cup quinoa, rinsed with hot water in a
    mesh strainer
2½ cups vegetable broth, low sodium
2 cups arugula, chopped
1 cup shitake mushrooms, thinly sliced
1 cup fresh or frozen peas (if frozen, thaw)
½ cup Parmesan cheese, freshly grated
Freshly ground black pepper to taste

Heat olive oil in a large nonstick saucepan over medium heat and sauté onion. Cook onions, stirring occasionally, on low to medium heat until onions are translucent, 4 to 5 minutes. Add the quinoa and stir for 1 minute. Add the vegetable broth, bring to a boil and then reduce heat to a simmer until quinoa is *al dente* (tender to the bite, but slightly hard in the center), 10 to 12 minutes.

Stir in the arugula, mushrooms and peas. Bring to a boil again, cover and simmer 5 to 8 minutes. Quinoa grains will turn translucent. Stir in the cheese and season with black pepper. Serve with a salad and fresh figs—if they're in season.

Traditionally risotto (from northern Italy) is made with rice, but I often like using quinoa because of its caviar-like texture and its high content of protein, vitamins and minerals, including zinc and iron.

Per serving (221 grams): 220 calories, 7.4 grams fat, 400 milligrams sodium, 28 grams carbohydrate, 4.1 grams dietary fiber, 12 grams protein.

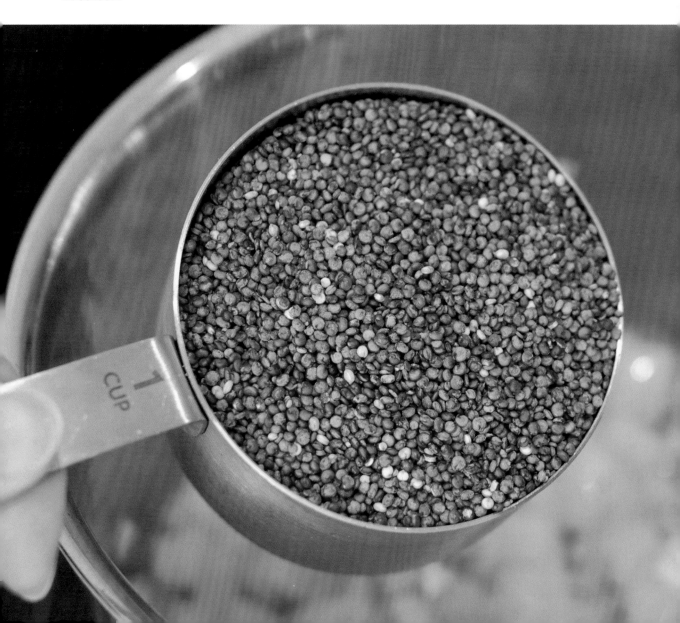

BAKED COD, SPINACH AND TOMATO IN FOIL PACKETS

Serves 4

1½ pounds cod fillets, about 1-inch thick
5 ounces fresh baby spinach
Freshly ground black pepper to taste
Freshly ground sea salt to taste (optional)
Citrus herb blend to taste (optional)
24 cherry tomatoes, cut in half
8 sprigs fresh thyme
1 lemon, cut into 4 wedges
1 tablespoon extra-virgin olive oil, divided

Preheat the oven to 400 degrees Fahrenheit.

Divide fish into four equal portions and remove any pin bones.

Lay out four sheets of aluminum foil, each about 12- to 14-inches long. Pile a handful of baby spinach leaves in the middle of each piece of foil.

Lay 1 fish fillet on each bed of spinach. According to your taste, season with black pepper and optional salt and/or citrus herb blend.

Scatter the cherry tomatoes on and around the fish. Lay 2 sprigs of thyme over each fillet. Give each packet a squeeze of lemon and a light sprinkle of olive oil.

Fold the sides of the foil inwards around the fish. Then, fold in the top and bottom of the foil and pinch them closed, creating a neat package. Set them side-by-side on a baking sheet and bake for 15 to 20 minutes, until the fish is opaque.

Open the packets carefully to avoid spilling the juices. Eat straight from the packets or transfer to a plate and serve with steamed green beans and a baked potato.

Optional: Add a splash of white wine over the fish before you seal the packets.

This is a no-mess, flavorful way to prepare seafood and veggies right at home. Cooking in the enclosed foil packets blends the flavors during baking, so there's hardly a pan to clean.

Per serving (578 grams): 270 calories, 5.8 grams fat, 44 milligrams sodium, 20 grams carbohydrates, 5.7 grams dietary fiber, 33 grams protein.

APRICOT GLAZED SALMON

Serves 4

1⅓ pounds salmon fillets (wild salmon when available)
¼ teaspoon freshly ground black pepper
1 tablespoon extra-virgin olive oil
1 clove garlic, minced
⅓ cup apricot fruit spread, 100 percent fruit
1 tablespoon Dijon mustard
½ cup low-sodium vegetable broth

Pat salmon dry with a paper towel and cut into four equal servings. Season the skinless side of salmon with pepper.

Heat oil in a large nonstick skillet on medium to high heat. Place salmon in skillet with skin side down.

Cook for 5 minutes and then turn fish over and cook another 5 minutes or until cooked through. Remove salmon to a plate and cover with foil to keep warm. Place garlic in the skillet and cook over medium heat for about 1 minute. Add remaining ingredients and stir.

Cook over medium heat for 3 to 5 minutes until ingredients and flavors are combined and glaze thickens. Pour glaze over salmon and serve over a bed of greens.

Salmon goes well with almost any grain. I like to serve such a rich-tasting fish with a hearty grain like brown rice. Salmon is high in omega-3 fatty acids, known for its natural anti-inflammatory effects.

Per serving (213 grams): 304 calories, 13 grams fat, 130 milligrams sodium, 14.3 grams carbohydrates, 30.4 grams protein.

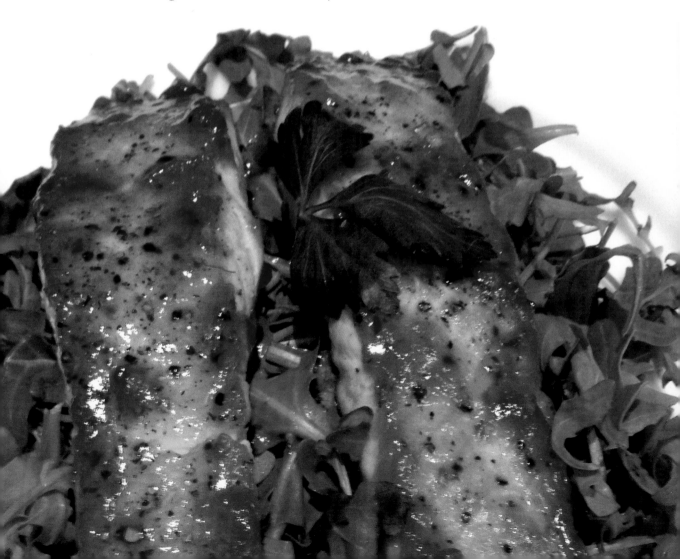

MEDITERRANEAN STEW

Serves 6

2 teaspoons extra-virgin olive oil
1 red onion, chopped
2 carrots, diced
3 plum tomatoes, chopped
5 ounces fresh baby spinach
2 cups water
1 cup uncooked whole-wheat couscous
26 ounces strained tomatoes
15 ounces chickpeas, canned, drained
    and rinsed
1 tablespoon fresh basil, chopped
½ teaspoon dried oregano (or
    1 tablespoon fresh)
Freshly ground black pepper to taste
Juice from 1 lemon (or 3 tablespoons fresh
    lemon juice)
Freshly grated Parmesan cheese to taste
    (optional)

Heat oil in a large nonstick saucepan on medium heat. Sauté onions until soft. Lower heat and add carrots and tomatoes; cook for 3 to 5 minutes. Add spinach, then water, couscous and strained tomatoes. Stir and then add chickpeas, basil, oregano, black pepper and lemon juice. Simmer uncovered for 10 to 15 minutes. Sprinkle with Parmesan cheese and serve with a mixed green salad.

This dish combines the protein of chickpeas with that of whole-wheat to make a complete protein, creating a perfectly balanced vegetarian plate.

Per serving (356 grams): 454 calories, 7.2 grams fat, 79 milligrams sodium, 81 grams carbohydrate, 18.6 grams dietary fiber, 21.5 grams protein.

SPRING FUSILLI WITH ASPARAGUS AND WALNUTS

Serves 4

8 ounces dry whole-wheat fusilli
1 pound fresh asparagus
2 tablespoons extra-virgin olive oil
1 clove garlic, minced
½ cup walnuts, chopped
Juice from 1 lemon (or 3 tablespoons fresh
    lemon juice)
1 teaspoon dried oregano (or
    1 tablespoon fresh)
½ cup flat-leaf parsley, chopped
¼ cup freshly grated Parmesan cheese
Freshly ground black pepper to taste

Cook pasta according to package directions and set aside. Trim off tough ends of asparagus and discard. Cut asparagus into 1-inch diagonal slices and set aside.

Heat oil in a large nonstick skillet over medium heat. Sauté garlic and asparagus for 3 minutes and add 2 tablespoons water if needed.

Add walnuts and cook 2 to 3 more minutes. Add pasta to skillet and then add lemon juice, oregano and parsley. Gently heat through and then sprinkle with Parmesan cheese and black pepper to taste. Serve with a citrus salad.

Asparagus is in season during the spring. You can enjoy this recipe year-round using mushrooms or a seasonal green vegetable of your choice.

Per serving (232 grams): 418 calories, 20.8 grams fat, 142 milligrams sodium, 43.4 grams carbohydrates, 9.3 grams dietary fiber, 18.7 grams protein.

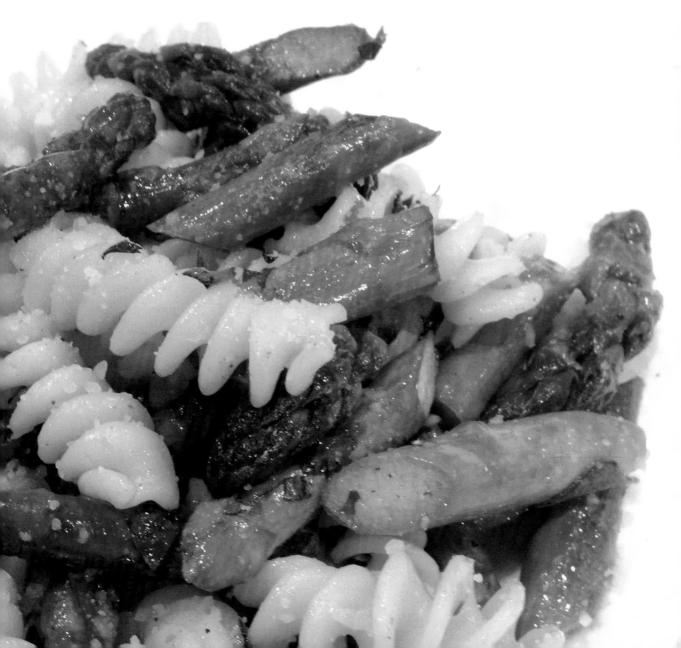

LONDON BROIL

Serves 6

(Requires marinating overnight)
2 pounds boneless top round "London
    broil" steak, about 2 inches thick
¼ cup balsamic vinegar
2 tablespoons extra-virgin olive oil
3 cloves garlic, crushed
1 teaspoon dried rosemary (or
    1 tablespoon fresh)
1 teaspoon dried thyme (or 1 tablespoon
    fresh)
Freshly ground black pepper to taste
Freshly ground sea salt to taste (optional)

In a small bowl, whisk together
vinegar, oil, garlic and herbs.

Place the beef on a cutting board
and poke both sides all over with a
fork. Transfer to a plastic freezer bag
and pour in the marinade. Seal and
refrigerate overnight.

Preheat oven on Broil, then remove
the London broil from the marinade
and pat dry. Season both sides with
pepper and optional salt. Place beef
on a broiler pan. Broil about eight
inches under the flame for 6 to 7
minutes per side for medium rare. The
internal temperature should reach
130 to 135 degrees Fahrenheit, or 55 to
57 degrees Celsius.

Transfer to a clean cutting board
and cover loosely with foil; let rest for
10 minutes. To serve, cut against the
grain into very thin slices. After slicing

meat, spoon any leftover juices over
sliced meat and serve over a bed of
arugula. Serve with steamed seasonal
vegetables and roasted new potatoes.

*London broil is not actually a cut of beef; it's
a method of preparing it. Because this dish is
made with top round steak, the leanest cut of
beef, slice it against the grain for maximum
tenderness. Buy grass-fed beef!*

Per serving (168 grams): 258 calories, 11.4 grams fat,
88 milligrams sodium, 0 carbohydrates, 34.9 grams protein.

CHICKEN, BROCCOLI AND COUSCOUS

Serves 4

1 tomato, chopped
1 tablespoon fresh basil, chopped
2 tablespoons balsamic vinegar
3 teaspoons extra-virgin olive oil, divided
1 clove garlic, minced
1 medium carrot, diced
1 pound boneless chicken breasts, cut into
    1-inch-wide strips
2 cups broccoli, chopped (discard thick
    stems)
1½ cups low-sodium chicken broth
1 cup uncooked couscous, preferably
    whole-wheat

Combine tomato, basil, vinegar and
1 teaspoon of oil and set aside. Heat
remaining 2 teaspoons of oil in a large

222

nonstick skillet on medium to high heat. Sauté garlic, carrot, chicken and broccoli for 5 to 6 minutes or until chicken is cooked thoroughly. Pour broth into skillet and bring to a boil. Add couscous, cover and remove from heat. Let stand 10 minutes. Divide tomato dressing evenly on four plates and then evenly plate chicken, broccoli and couscous. Fluff the couscous with a fork as you serve it.

This dish is the perfect one-pot meal!

Per serving (319 grams): 390 calories, 7.4 grams fat, 118 milligrams sodium, 37.7 grams carbohydrates, 3.5 grams dietary fiber, 40.6 grams protein.

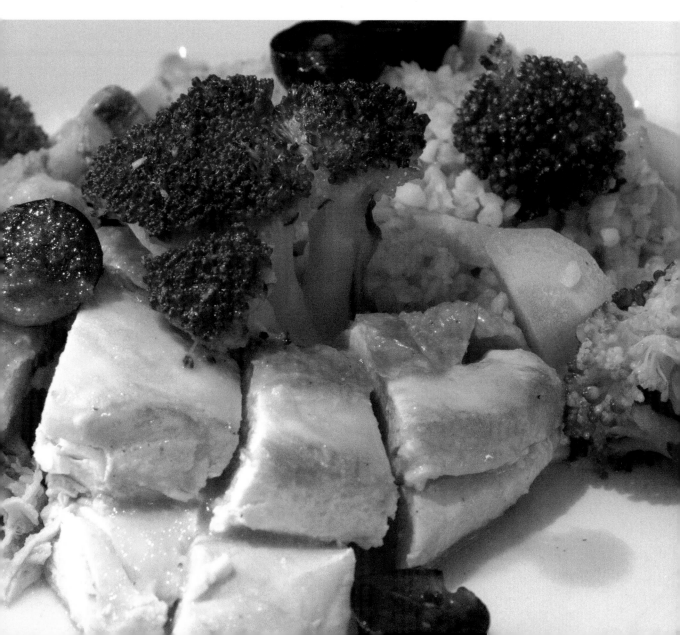

SPINACH LASAGNA

Serves 10

32 ounces part-skim or lite ricotta cheese

12 ounces silken firm tofu, drained

1 tablespoon dried Italian seasoning (a
    mix of oregano, basil and parsley or
    2 tablespoons fresh Italian herbs)

52 ounces no-salt-added tomato sauce
    (homemade or jarred)

8 ounces lasagna noodles, preferably
    whole-wheat (or 9 noodles)

5 ounces baby spinach

1 cup part-skim mozzarella cheese,
    shredded

Preheat oven to 350 degrees Fahrenheit.
Place ricotta, tofu and Italian
seasoning in a food processor and
blend on high speed. In a 9-inch by
12-inch pan, layer lasagna in this order:
sauce, three lasagna noodles, ricotta
filling and spinach. Repeat this two
more times and end with sauce on top,
then sprinkle with mozzarella cheese.
Cover the lasagna with foil and bake
for 1 hour or until heated through and
pasta is tender. Allow lasagna to stand
for 10 minutes, and then cut into 10
cubes. Serve with a mixed green salad.

*There is no need to pre-cook lasagna
noodles when this much sauce is used in the
preparation. You can decrease the sauce to
48 ounces, and then add a total of 4 ounces
of water to the jars of the sauce. Swish it
around, and pour it along the outsides of the
dish before baking.*

Per serving (333 grams): 350 calories, 15 grams fat, 340
milligrams sodium, 34 grams carbohydrates, 5.1 grams dietary
fiber, 23.2 grams protein.

TURKEY BREAST MEATBALLS

Serves 5

3 egg whites, lightly beaten

½ cup onions, finely chopped

1¼ pounds ground turkey breast meat only

½ cup Parmesan cheese, freshly grated

2 tablespoons fresh flat-leaf parsley, finely
    chopped

¼ teaspoon garlic powder

½ cup plain, dry breadcrumbs

1 teaspoon freshly ground black pepper

1½ teaspoons garlic clove, minced

1 tablespoon dried oregano (or
    2 tablespoons fresh)

1 tablespoon dried basil (or 2 tablespoons
    fresh)

Preheat oven to 450 degrees Fahrenheit.
In a large bowl, thoroughly combine
all ingredients. With clean, wet hands,
form mixture into 10 meatballs by
rolling between the palms of your
hands. Place meatballs in a large
baking pan with a small amount of
water—just enough to coat the pan.

Cook for 20 minutes or until done. Keep an eye on the pan and add water if needed. Serve with your favorite tomato sauce over whole-grain pasta and steamed escarole.

Leave out the cheese if you prefer dairy-free meatballs.

Per serving of two meatballs (182 grams): 258 calories, 6 grams fat, 380 milligrams sodium, 11.2 grams carbohydrates, 39.6 grams protein.

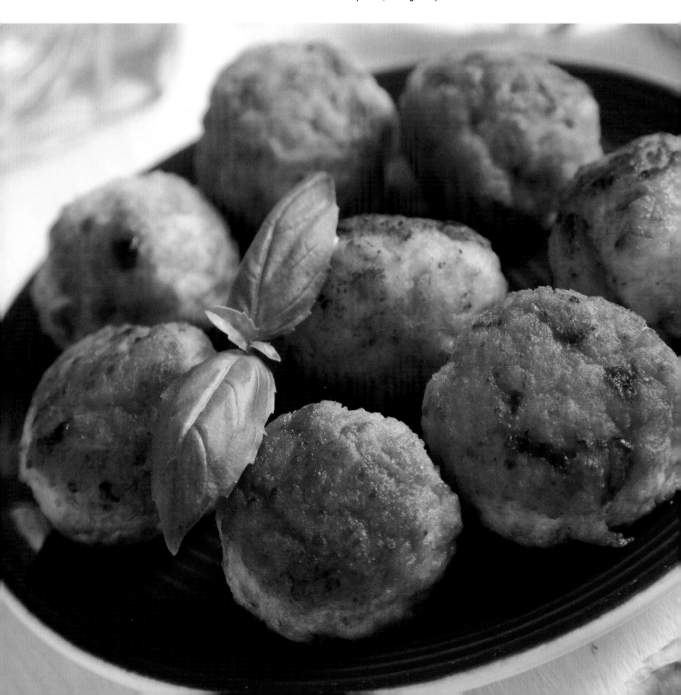

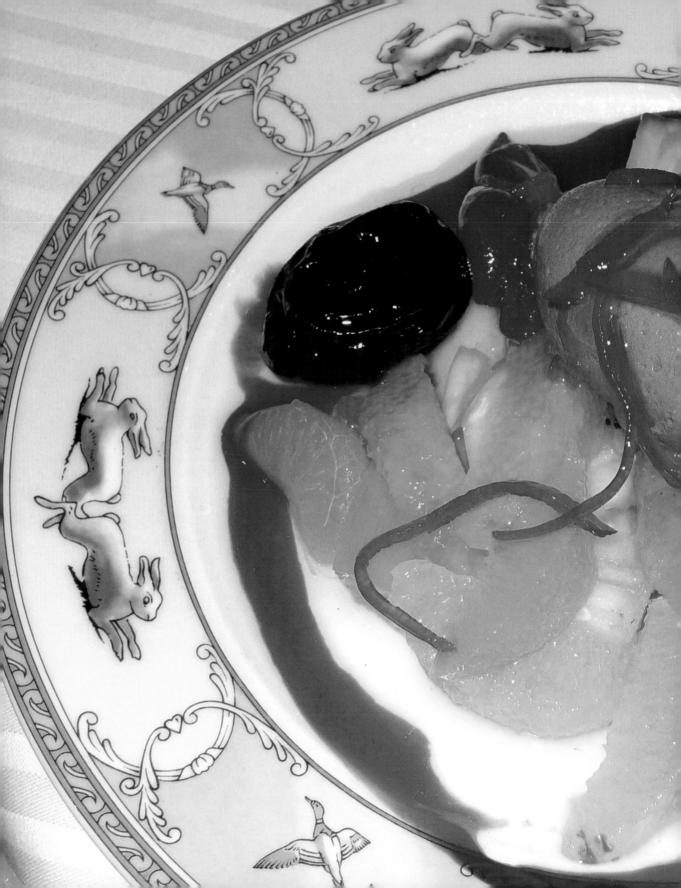

PAUL BOCUSE

Chapter 14

DREAMY DESSERTS AND FABULOUS FINALES

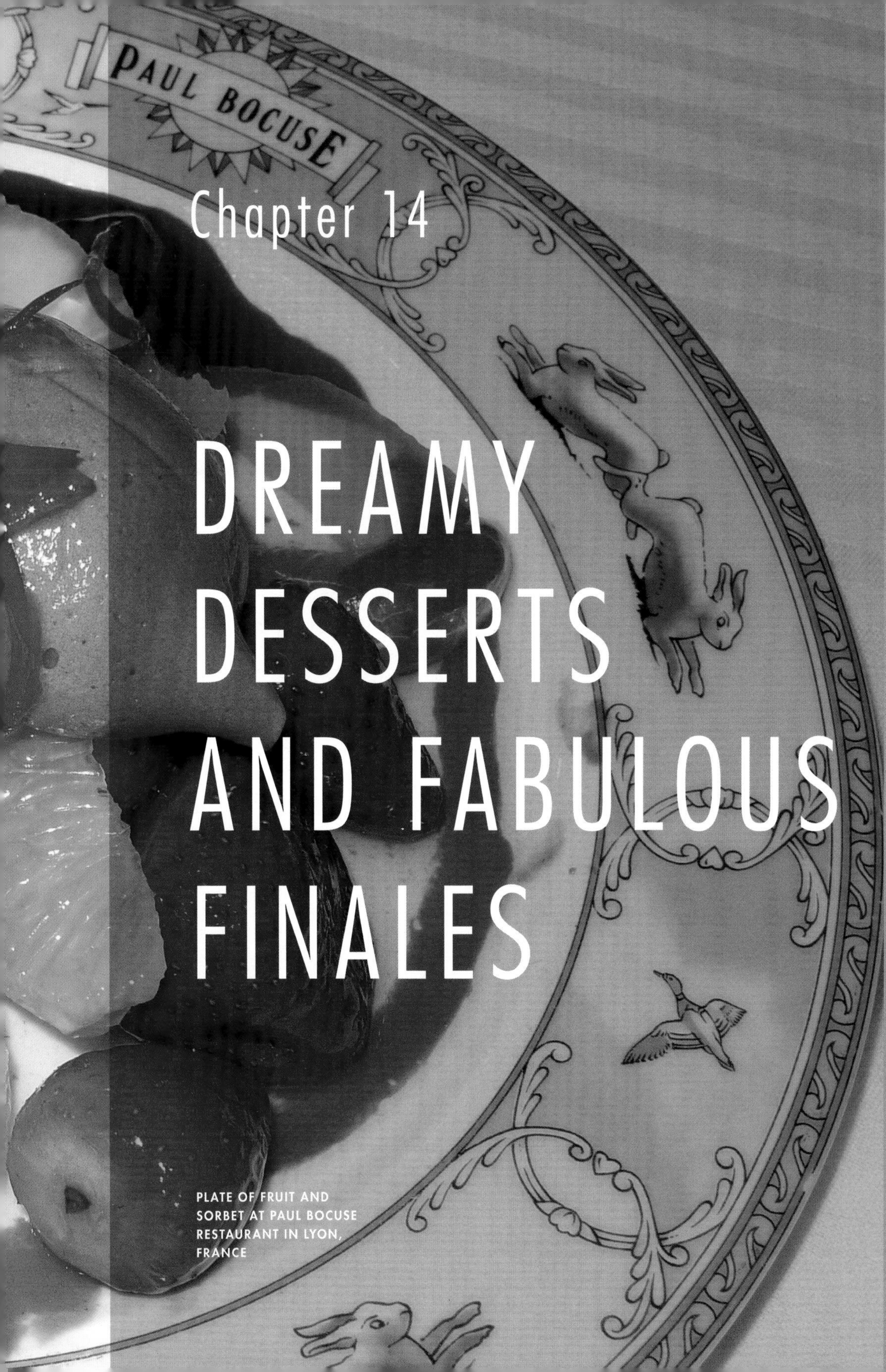

PLATE OF FRUIT AND
SORBET AT PAUL BOCUSE
RESTAURANT IN LYON,
FRANCE

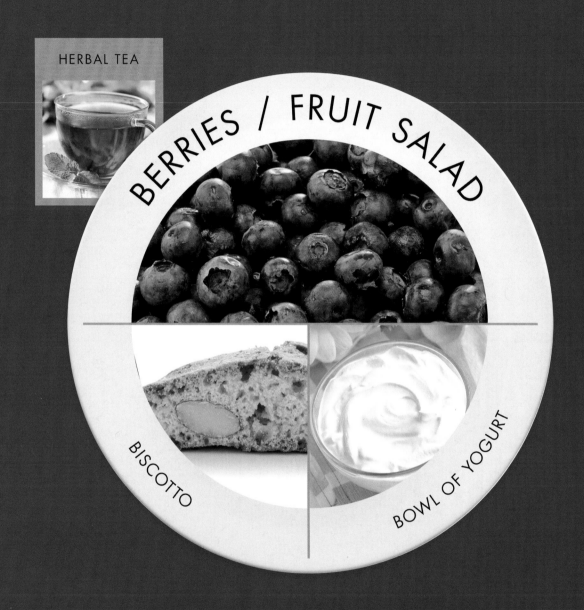

HERBAL TEA

BERRIES / FRUIT SALAD

BISCOTTO

BOWL OF YOGURT

SUPER-HEALTHY DESSERT PLATE GUIDE

At home, Europeans favor fruit-filled desserts, including pastries stuffed with seasonal fruit that aren't overly sweet. Often, dessert will consist of fresh, dried or cooked fruit served with aged or fresh cheese. Chocolate (preferably dark) also takes center stage and enjoys top ratings, along with fine wine and cheese.

Chocolate lovers, feel free to splurge on high-quality cocoa powder, which gives you the chocolate flavor without all the calories and fat found in other forms of chocolate! Cocoa powder has no added sugar, only 12 grams of fat, and 196 calories per cup and is the perfect base for a rich cup of hot cocoa or a delicious mousse. It's also an excellent source of potassium and contains choline, folic acid and lutein, all of which benefit your nervous system, skin and vision.

Chocolate contains caffeine, so consider having your fix in the afternoon and stick to fruit in the evening. Since it's the cocoa bean that contains the caffeine, the higher the percentage of cocoa in the chocolate, the higher the caffeine content. One cup of dry, unsweetened cocoa powder has about 200 milligrams of caffeine—that's 25 milligrams per ounce. A 1-ounce square of unsweetened baking chocolate contains 23 milligrams of caffeine. Hot cocoa averages 10 milligrams of caffeine per 8-ounce cup, which is much less than the 102 to 200 milligrams found in an 8-ounce cup of brewed coffee.

For those sensitive to caffeine's effects—it can raise blood pressure and heart rate—it's best to avoid both coffee and chocolate.

If you have an insatiable sweet craving, take the edge off with a cup of herbal tea, such as chamomile, carob or mint, wait it out, take a walk and then enjoy a piece of fruit. Or you can try these healthy dessert recipes created just for you!

DESSERT RECIPES

LADYFINGER CAKE WITH MIXED BERRY MARNIER (GLUTEN-FREE, NO ADDED FAT)

Serves 6

3 egg whites
½ teaspoon cream of tartar
⅓ cup organic sugar
1 teaspoon vanilla extract
¼ teaspoon baking powder
½ cup all-purpose, gluten-free baking flour
Nonstick cooking spray, olive oil

For Berries:

1½ cups fresh mixed berries
1 navel orange, juice only
2 tablespoons Grand Marnier brandy
    liqueur

Bring eggs to room temperature for 30 minutes and preheat oven to 350 degrees Fahrenheit. Spray a shallow 6- or 8-inch round baking dish with nonstick cooking spray. In a glass or stainless steel bowl, beat eggs (using a hand mixer or whisk) until frothy, and then add cream of tartar and mix until soft peaks form. Beat in the sugar a little at a time until stiffer peaks form. Slowly fold in the vanilla, baking powder, and flour, and then slowly pour the batter into the pan. Bake for 20 minutes until the cake is golden brown and a toothpick inserted in the middle comes out clean. The sides of the cake will also pull away from the pan.

While the cake is baking, prepare the berries: In a large bowl, combine the berries, orange juice and Grand Marnier. Allow the berries to sit at room temperature for at least 1 hour and stir periodically. If the berries are not sweet enough, add ½ teaspoon of sugar.

Allow the cake to cool upside down for 10 to 20 minutes. Run a knife around the edge of the cake and turn it out onto a cake plate. Cut into oblong pieces or whatever shapes you desire. Evenly divide the fruit and spoon over the cake; serve.

Use this cake as a replacement for sponge cake in any recipe. It works well for a tiramisu. Use cognac or any other fruit brandy as a substitute for Grand Marnier.

Per serving (138 grams): 150 calories, 0.7 grams fat, 28 milligrams sodium, 29.7 grams carbohydrates, 3.1 grams dietary fiber, 3.5 grams protein.

MARINATED FRESH FRUIT SALAD

Serves 4

3 cups fresh fruit, chopped
¼ cup white wine
Juice of 2 oranges
2 teaspoons lemon juice
1 tablespoon honey or agave syrup

$\frac{1}{16}$ teaspoon (or a pinch) ground cloves
$\frac{1}{8}$ teaspoon ground cinnamon

In a large bowl, combine fruit with rest of ingredients. Chill and serve.

Create your own combinations of seasonal fruit salad. In winter, add dried fruit to chopped citrus and sliced banana. For crunch in any fruit salad, add chopped walnuts. If you prefer to leave out the wine, replace it with freshly squeezed orange juice.

Per serving without nuts (224 grams): 115 calories, 0 fat, 25 milligrams sodium, 26 grams carbohydrates, 1.3 grams dietary fiber, 1.5 grams protein.

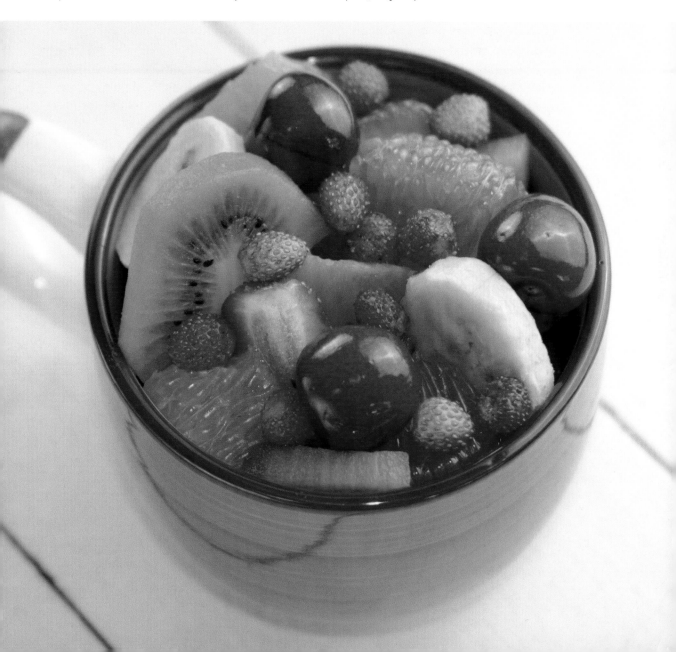

RHUBARB AND STRAWBERRY COMPOTE

Serves 6

6 large stalks rhubarb
1 cup strawberries, stems removed, diced
¼ cup pure maple syrup
Water to "almost" cover rhubarb
4 cubes crystallized ginger, chopped
¼ teaspoon ground cinnamon (or to taste)

Cut off tough ends of rhubarb and discard ends. Cut remaining rhubarb into bite-size pieces. Place rhubarb in a large non-reactive saucepan and pour in a small amount of water to barely cover the rhubarb. Add maple syrup and ginger.

Bring to boil and then lower heat to a simmer for 10 minutes, stirring occasionally. Add strawberries during the last 2 minutes of cooking. Season with ground cinnamon. Rhubarb will soften and become stringy. Allow it to cool and then strain liquid or use it as part of the dessert. (I prefer to use it.) Serve with optional whipped cream.

Rhubarb contains vitamins A and C, calcium and potassium. It's versatile and easy to grow in your garden or in a pot.

Per serving (155 grams): 124 calories, 0 fat, 7 milligrams sodium, 30.3 grams carbohydrates, 1.3 grams dietary fiber, 0.6 gram protein.

POACHED PEARS

Serves 4

4 firm-ripe pears, cored and sliced in half
¼ cup water
¼ cup white wine (sweet or dry) or sparkling cider
¼ cup pure maple syrup
½ teaspoon ground cinnamon

Preheat oven to 350 degrees Fahrenheit.

In a large bowl, combine pears with water and white wine. Add syrup and cinnamon and stir until fruit is evenly coated. Spoon into an 8-inch square glass baking dish. Bake 20 to 30 minutes or until pears are tender. Serve warm with sorbet or tart frozen yogurt.

Use any seasonal variety of pears: Bartlett, bosc, comice, forelle and anjou are just a few.

Pears are a favorite fruit of the French and are a good source of antioxidants, dietary fiber, immune-supporting vitamin-C and bone-building vitamin K.

Per serving (259 grams): 186 calories, 0 fat, 5 milligrams sodium, 46 grams carbohydrates, 6.6 grams dietary fiber, 1 gram protein.

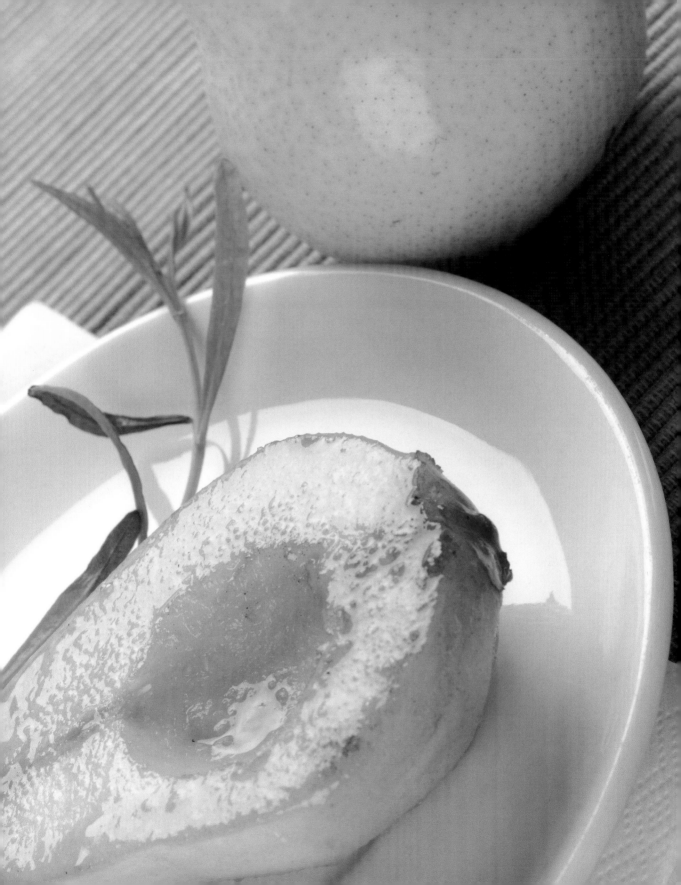

APPLE WALNUT CAKE

Serves 6

1 cup whole-wheat graham flour or flour
   of your choice
¼ cup organic sugar
¾ teaspoon double-acting baking powder
½ teaspoon ground cinnamon
1/16 teaspoon (or a pinch) ground nutmeg
¼ teaspoon salt
1 large apple, finely chopped
½ cup walnuts, finely chopped
1 egg or 2 egg whites
½ cup unsweetened apple juice
½ cup unsweetened applesauce
Nonstick cooking spray, olive oil

Preheat oven to 350 degrees Fahrenheit.
   In a medium-sized bowl, combine
flour, sugar, baking powder, spices and
salt. In another medium-sized bowl,
combine apples and walnuts. Lightly
dust apples and walnuts with a small
amount of the flour mixture. In a third
large bowl, lightly beat egg or egg
whites, apple juice and applesauce.
Add flour mixture to the egg mixture.
Mix well, then gently fold apple and
chopped walnuts into batter. Spray
a nonstick 8-inch by 4-inch loaf pan
(or 6-inch by 2-inch round pan) with
cooking spray. Turn batter into pan.
Bake for 30 to 35 minutes or until
toothpick comes out clean. It's not
overly sweet and pairs well with a
scoop of vanilla frozen yogurt.

*This cake is also delicious at breakfast and
with afternoon tea.*

*"An apple a day keeps the doctor away" is
one of those sayings that has lots of truth to
it, so add another apple if you like it fruity!*

*Walnuts have beneficial heart-healthy
vitamin E and omega 3 fatty acids.*

Per serving made with a whole egg (125 grams):
210 calories, 7 grams fat, 160 milligrams sodium, 34 grams
carbohydrates, 4.6 grams dietary fiber, 5.5 grams protein.

CHOCOLATE TOFU MOUSSE

Serves 10

14 ounces firm tofu, silken preferred
½ cup agave syrup, honey or pure
   maple syrup
¾ cup cocoa powder
2 teaspoons vanilla extract

Place tofu in a blender or food
processor and blend until smooth.
Place sweetener in a small bowl and
heat in microwave for 30 seconds. Add
cocoa powder to the hot sweetener
and stir until smooth. Pour the sweet
cocoa syrup and vanilla into the
blender and blend with the tofu. Pour
into a pie pan and chill for 4 hours or
overnight. Garnish with fresh fruit
before serving.

This is a rich dessert, and if made with good quality cocoa powder, a few spoonfuls will satisfy even the most discerning chocolate connoisseur.

If you are avoiding caffeine, substitute carob powder for the cocoa powder. Carob comes from the pod of a tree that grows along the Mediterranean coast. The pulp from the pod is ground into a powder, creating carob powder.

Per serving with agave syrup (80 grams): 112 calories, 2.4 grams fat, 19 milligrams sodium, 21.7 grams carbohydrates, 2.4 grams dietary fiber, 4.9 grams protein.

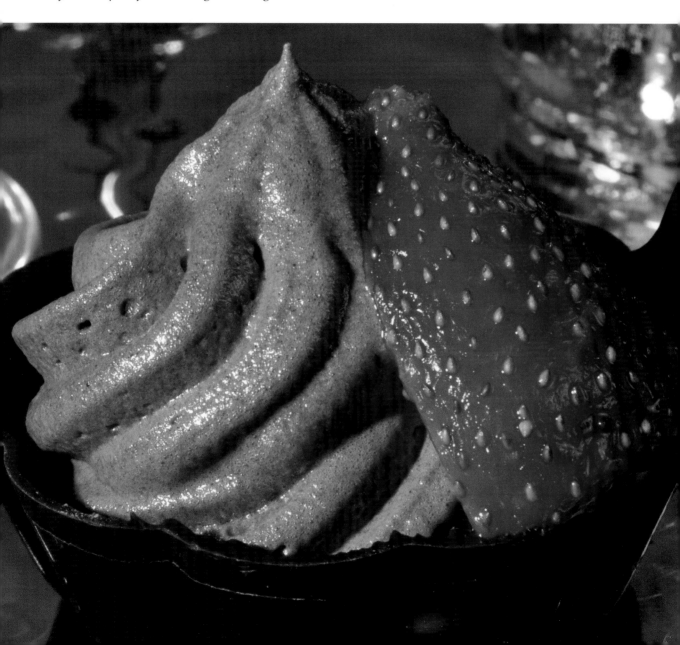

RICOTTA CHEESECAKE (CRUSTLESS) WITH BERRIES

Serves 6

2 cups part-skim or lite ricotta cheese
1 tablespoon unbleached, all-purpose flour
1 egg plus 2 egg whites, beaten
⅓ cup honey or agave syrup
1 teaspoon vanilla extract
Nonstick cooking spray, olive oil
3 cups mixed frozen berries, thawed

Preheat oven to 350 degrees Fahrenheit.

In a blender, combine all ingredients except berries until smooth. Spray a 6-inch by 2-inch (or 8-inch by 1½-inch) round pan with nonstick cooking spray. Spoon the mixture into the pan and level the top.

Bake for 1 hour or until set and golden on top. Allow to cool.

Meanwhile, to make the berry sauce, place the berries in a medium saucepan and heat on low until softened. If the berries are tart, add your choice of natural sweetener, 1 teaspoon at a time. Cool and serve with sliced ricotta cheesecake.

If you prefer a flourless cake, then leave out the flour—it works well with or without flour.

Per serving made with part-skim ricotta and berries included (188 grams): 208 calories, 7 grams fat, 143 milligrams sodium, 29 grams carbohydrates, 2.6 grams dietary fiber, 10.8 grams protein.

YOGURT PANNA COTTA

Serves 4

2 teaspoons unflavored gelatin or powdered agar agar
½ cup fat-free milk or original almond milk
1 tablespoon honey or agave syrup
12 ounces nonfat Greek vanilla yogurt
1 teaspoon pure vanilla extract
1 cup fresh berries or diced seasonal fruit (for garnish)

In a small microwave-safe bowl, sprinkle the gelatin or agar agar over the milk and let stand for 5 minutes. After gelatin (or agar agar) has softened, heat the mixture in the microwave for 30 seconds. Stir to make sure the gelatin (or agar agar) is dissolved. If not dissolved, heat for 3 seconds more and stir again.

In a separate medium bowl, whisk together the honey or agave, yogurt, vanilla extract and milk/gelatin (or agar agar) mixture.

Divide the mixture among four (½ cup) ramekins or custard cups. Cover and chill overnight. Before serving, garnish with berries or fruit of your choice.

Agar agar is a vegetarian gelling agent made from algae. The powdered form works well as a substitute for gelatin.

Per serving with berries (156 grams): 113 calories, 0 fat, 68 milligrams sodium, 18.6 grams carbohydrates, 1.8 grams dietary fiber, 9.8 grams protein.

236

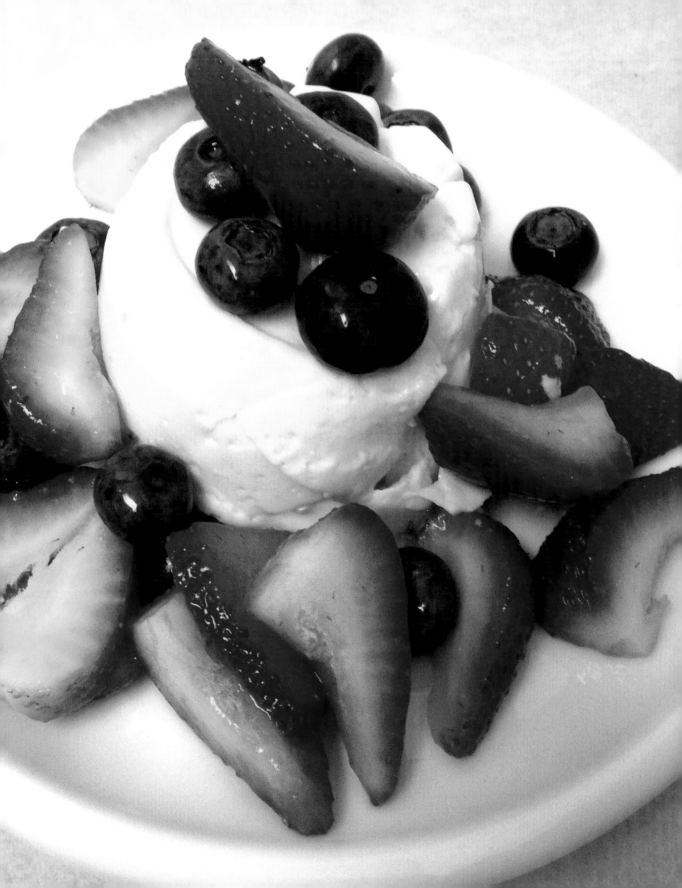

BAKED APPLES WITH CRANBERRIES AND PISTACHIOS

Serves 4

4 apples (your favorite variety), cored and
    cut into ½-inch slices
⅓ cup natural cranberry juice, or
    unsweetened apple juice
½ cup dried cranberries
¼ cup unsalted pistachio nuts
1 teaspoon ground cinnamon

Preheat oven to 350 degrees Fahrenheit.
    Place sliced apples in a medium
baking dish. Drizzle juice over apples.
Sprinkle cranberries, pistachio nuts
and cinnamon over the top. Bake 20 to
30 minutes or until apples are tender.
(Check the apples during cooking and
add ¼ cup water if needed.)

*If you don't have dried cranberries on hand,
try this recipe with your favorite dried
fruit (chopped). Alternatively, substitute
pecans or candied pecans (chopped) for the
pistachios.*

Per serving (226 grams): 159 calories, 3.6 grams fat,
4 milligrams sodium, 32.4 grams carbohydrates, 6 grams
dietary fiber, 1.8 grams protein.

ROASTED FIGS

Serves 4

12 fresh figs, cut in half
2 tablespoons balsamic vinegar
Nonstick cooking spray, olive oil

Preheat oven to 400 degrees Fahrenheit.
    Line a baking sheet with foil and
spray foil with nonstick cooking
spray. Place halved figs on foil or
directly on a medium-sized roasting
pan. Evenly drizzle with vinegar.
Roast for 8 to 10 minutes or until
bubbly on top. If you plan to serve
figs as an accompaniment to poultry
or lean meat, add a few sprigs of
fresh rosemary to the roasting pan.
Dried cranberries, toasted pistachios
and slivered almonds are optional
garnishes.

*Figs are in season early summer and early
fall, so enjoy them while they last!*

*In winter, when fresh figs are out of season,
buy dried figs and soak them in water
overnight in the fridge. Chop and serve
on top of cereal, yogurt and salad or as an
accompaniment to poultry, meat and fish.*

Per serving for 3 large figs (192 grams): 135 calories, 0 fat,
0 sodium, 36 grams carbohydrates, 6 grams dietary fiber,
3 grams protein.

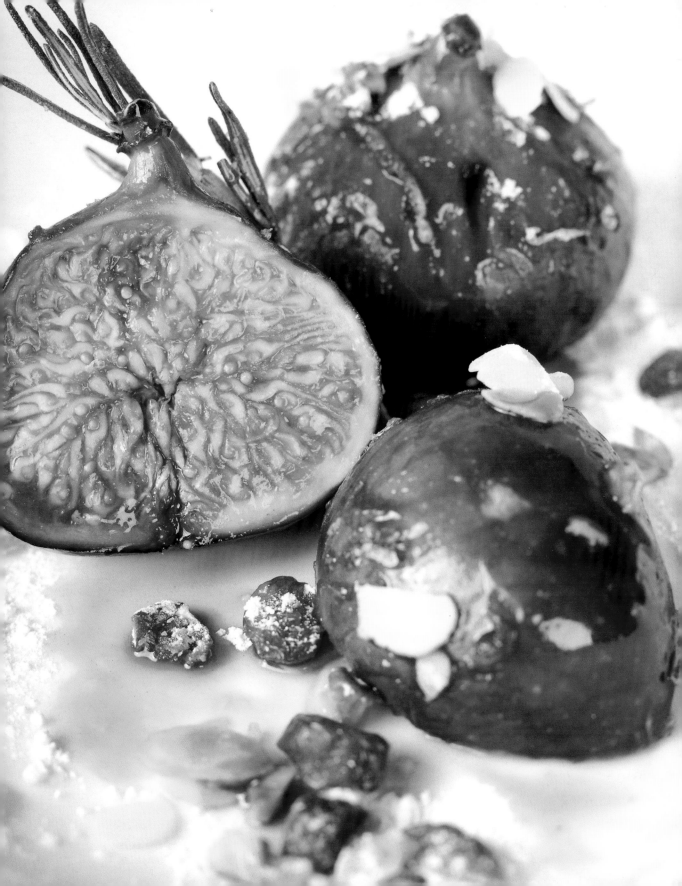

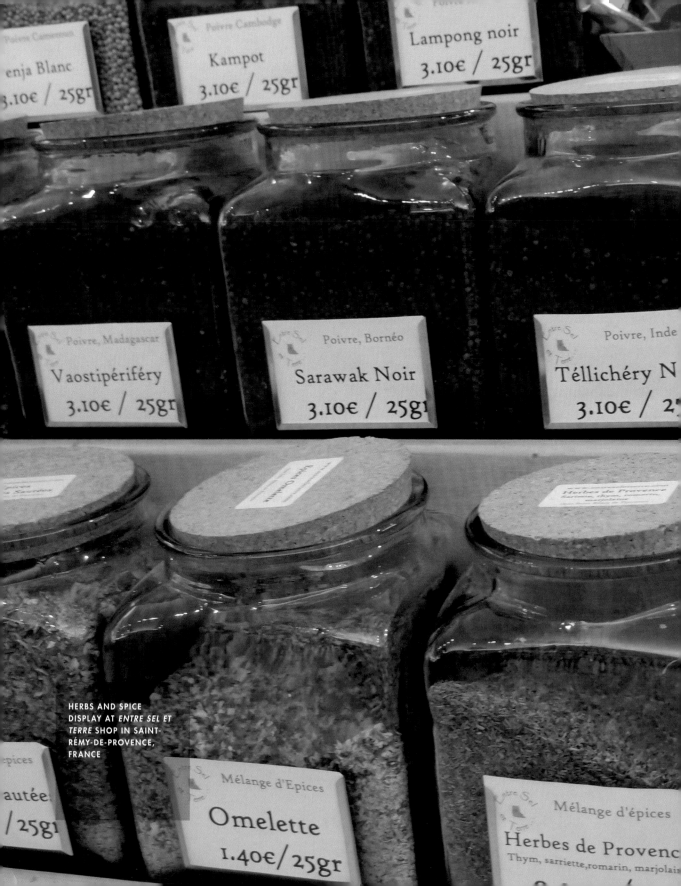

enja Blanc
3.10€ / 25gr

Poivre Cameroun

Kampot
3.10€ / 25gr

Poivre Cambodge

Lampong noir
3.10€ / 25gr

Poivre, Madagascar
Vaostipériféry
3.10€ / 25gr

Poivre, Bornéo
Sarawak Noir
3.10€ / 25gr

Poivre, Inde
Téllichéry N
3.10€ / 2

HERBS AND SPICE
DISPLAY AT *ENTRE SEL ET
TERRE* SHOP IN SAINT-
RÉMY-DE-PROVENCE,
FRANCE

épices
a Sautée

Mélange d'Epices
Omelette
1.40€/25gr

Mélange d'épices
Herbes de Provence
Thym, sarriette, romarin, marjolai

APPENDIX

COMPARISON OF DIETARY FATS

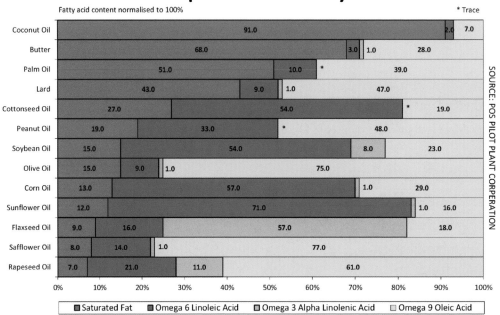

Comparison of Dietary Fats

Fatty acid content normalised to 100%   * Trace

Oil	Saturated Fat	Omega 6 Linoleic Acid	Omega 3 Alpha Linolenic Acid	Omega 9 Oleic Acid
Coconut Oil	91.0		2.0	7.0
Butter	68.0	3.0	1.0	28.0
Palm Oil	51.0	10.0	*	39.0
Lard	43.0	9.0	1.0	47.0
Cottonseed Oil	27.0	54.0	*	19.0
Peanut Oil	19.0	33.0	*	48.0
Soybean Oil	15.0	54.0	8.0	23.0
Olive Oil	15.0	9.0	1.0	75.0
Corn Oil	13.0	57.0	1.0	29.0
Sunflower Oil	12.0	71.0	1.0	16.0
Flaxseed Oil	9.0	16.0	57.0	18.0
Safflower Oil	8.0	14.0	1.0	77.0
Rapeseed Oil	7.0	21.0	11.0	61.0

0% 10% 20% 30% 40% 50% 60% 70% 80% 90% 100%

■ Saturated Fat   ■ Omega 6 Linoleic Acid   □ Omega 3 Alpha Linolenic Acid   □ Omega 9 Oleic Acid

SOURCE: POS PILOT PLANT CORPERATION

Note that omega-9 oleic acid is a monounsaturated fat. Omega-6 and omega-3 fatty acids are polyunsaturated fats.

Source: http://www.hillfarmoils.com

HOW TO READ FOOD NUTRITION LABELS

In addition to the Nutrition Facts label, many foods today come with nutrient content claims provided by the manufacturer. These claims are typically featured in ads for the foods or in the promotional copy on the food packages themselves. The U.S. Food and Drug Administration (FDA) strictly defines them. The chart below provides some of the most commonly used nutrient content claims, along with a detailed description of what the claim means.

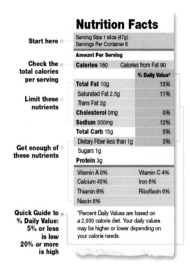

If a food claims to be...	It means that one serving of the product contains...
Calorie free	Less than 5 calories
Sugar free	Less than 0.5 grams of sugar
Fat	
Fat free	Less than 0.5 grams of fat
Low fat	3 grams of fat or less
Reduced fat or less fat	At least 25 percent less fat than the regular product
Low in saturated fat	1 gram of saturated fat or less, with not more than 15 percent of the calories coming from saturated fat
Lean	Less than 10 grams of fat, 4.5 grams of saturated fat and 95 milligrams of cholesterol
Extra lean	Less than 5 grams of fat, 2 grams of saturated fat and 95 milligrams of cholesterol
Light (lite)	At least one-third fewer calories or no more than half the fat of the regular product, or no more than half the sodium of the regular product
Cholesterol	
Cholesterol free	Less than 2 milligrams of cholesterol and 2 grams (or less) of saturated fat
Low cholesterol	20 or fewer milligrams of cholesterol and 2 grams or less of saturated fat
Reduced cholesterol	At least 25 percent less cholesterol than the regular product and 2 grams or less of saturated fat
Sodium	
Sodium free or no sodium	Less than 5 milligrams of sodium and no sodium chloride in ingredients
Very low sodium	35 milligrams or less of sodium
Low sodium	140 milligrams or less of sodium
Reduced or less sodium	At least 25 percent less sodium than the regular product
Fiber	
High fiber	5 grams or more of fiber
Good source of fiber	2.5 to 4.9 grams of fiber

243

If you can't remember the definitions of all of the terms, don't worry. You can use these general guidelines instead:

"Free" means a food has the least possible amount of the specified nutrient.

"Very Low" and "Low" means the food has a little more than foods labeled "Free."

"Reduced" or "Less" mean the food has 25 percent less of a specific nutrient than the regular version of the food.

Source: The American Heart Association

HOW MANY SERVINGS OF EACH FOOD GROUP DO I NEED FOR CALORIE CONTROL?

Here are the suggested number of servings from each food group based on consuming 1,500 and 2,000 calories per day. Calorie needs depend on age, weight, height, physical activity and whether you are trying to lose, gain or maintain weight. If you need fewer calories than 1,500, decrease the number of servings; if you need more than 1,500 calories, increase the servings.

Calories	*About 1,500*	*About 2,000*
Grain/Starchy Group	*7 servings*	*9 servings*
Vegetable Group	*At least 3 servings*	*At least 4 servings*
Fruit Group	*3 servings*	*4 servings*
Milk/Dairy Alternatives Group	*2 to 3 servings*	*3 servings*
Protein Group	*4 servings*	*6 servings*
Fats/Sweets	*3 servings*	*4 servings*

WHAT COUNTS AS ONE SERVING?

Here is a serving size guide to help you with what counts as one serving for each food group. For example, one cup of cooked pasta equals two servings of grain/starch.

Fats, Oils & Sweets:
Limit calories from this group especially if trying to lose weight. Choose monounsaturated fat like extra-virgin olive oil. Try cocoa or 1 ounce of dark chocolate to satisfy a sweet tooth (>70 percent cocoa). One teaspoon of oil or 2 teaspoons of jam equals one serving.

Milk, Yogurt and Dairy Alternatives Group:
1 cup low-fat milk or yogurt, 1 cup enriched almond, rice, oat or soy milk

Protein Group (Meat, Poultry, Fish, Beans, Eggs, Nuts, Cheese):
1 ounce cooked extra-lean meat, poultry or fish, ¼ cup cooked beans, 2 teaspoons natural peanut butter, 1 egg, 3 egg whites, 4 ounces tofu, 1 ounce low fat cheese, 2 tablespoons part skim ricotta

Fruit Group:
1 fresh fruit, ½ cup canned fruit/applesauce, 2 tablespoons dried fruit, ½ cup freshly squeezed fruit juice

Vegetable Group:
½ cup cooked non-starchy vegetables, 1 cup leafy greens or salad, ½ cup vegetable juice

Grain & Starch Group:
1 slice whole-grain bread, ½ English muffin, ½ cup cooked brown rice/pasta/grain, ½ cup cooked muesli or oatmeal, 1 ounce of ready-to-eat cereal, 1 ear corn, 3-ounce potato

WHAT TO STOCK IN YOUR PANTRY/FREEZER

Select Organic Ingredients When Available

Whole-Wheat/All-Purpose Flour

Oats/Cornmeal

Whole-Grain Pasta

Whole-Wheat Couscous/Quinoa

Baking Powder/Baking Soda

Brown/Wild Rice

Rice/Wasa Crackers

Organic Sugar/Coconut Sugar

Sea Salt/Salt Blends

Canned Tomatoes

Walnuts/Dry-Roasted Almonds

Assorted Dried Herbs:
   Oregano/Basil/Rosemary/Parsley/Thyme

Frozen Spinach/Kale

Frozen Shrimp

Pure Maple Syrup

Raw Honey/Black Strap Molasses

   (DO NOT GIVE RAW HONEY TO

   INFANTS UNDER THE AGE OF ONE)

Dijon Mustard/Ketchup

Unsweetened Cocoa Powder

Canned Beans, Organic

Cold-Pressed, Extra-Virgin Olive Oil

Balsamic Vinegar

Low-Sodium Chicken/Vegetable Broth, Organic

Ground Cinnamon/Nutmeg/Vanilla Extract

White/Black/Pink Peppercorns/
   Espelette Pepper

Frozen Peas/Corn

Apricot Jam/Mango Chutney

Natural Nut Butter	*Dried Lentils/Beans*
Dried Cranberries/Prunes/Dates	*Pumpkin Seeds*
Unsweetened Applesauce/Apple juice	*Original Almond Milk*
Tomato Sauce/Strained Tomatoes	*Tofu*

CALORIES IN ALCOHOLIC BEVERAGES

It's easy to forget that you can drink as many calories as you eat. In fact, some drinks can have as many calories as a meal! Calories in wine and beer will vary depending on the content of alcohol. Those with a higher alcohol content will contain more calories. Remember to check the serving size and to add the calories from any juice or mixer that is combined with the liquor.

Alcoholic Drink	Average Calories	Alcoholic Drink	Average Calories
Beer, lite, 12 oz.	100	Whiskey, 1.5 oz.	105
Beer, regular, 12 oz.	150	Wine, red, 4 oz.	100
Frozen daiquiri, 4 oz.	216	Wine, white, 4 oz.	100
Gin, 1.5 oz.	110	Champagne, 4 oz.	80
Mai tai, 4 oz.	310	Prosecco, 4 oz.	80
Margarita, 4 oz.	270	Wine spritzer, 4 oz.	49
Rum, 1.5 oz.	96	Wine, dessert, sweet, 4 oz.	180
Vodka, 1.5 oz.	96		

Adapted from: http://www.medicinenet.com/alcohol_and_nutrition/page3.htm

ORGANIC, SUSTAINABLE AND BIODYNAMIC WINE: WHICH ONE IS BEST FOR YOU?

There's been alarming news that many wines and spirits, even those imported from Europe, are showing up with high pesticide counts. Luckily, there are choices, and you can read here about the differences between organic, biodynamic and sustainable wines. These practices of production vary in the way they're defined and regulated, so here is an explanation of how they're most typically defined.

The U.S. government regulates the use of the term "organic," but "sustainable" and "biodynamic" have no legal definitions.

Organic: There are two types of organic listings on wine bottles. Wines can be made from certified organically grown grapes, avoiding any synthetic additives. Or to take it a step further, "organic" wines are made from organically grown grapes and are also made without any added sulfites—though naturally occurring sulfites will still be present.

Biodynamic: It is similar to organic farming in that both take place without synthetic chemicals, but biodynamic farming incorporates ideas about a vineyard as an eco-system, and also accounts for astrological influences and lunar cycles. A biodynamic wine means that the grapes are farmed biodynamically, and that the winemaker did not make the wine with any common manipulations such as yeast additions or acid-ity adjustments. A wine "made from biodynamic grapes" means that a vintner used biodynamically grown grapes, but followed a less strict list of "rules" in winemaking.

Sustainable: This incorporates a range of practices that are not only ecologically sound, but also economically viable and socially responsible. Sustainable farmers may farm largely organically or biodynamically but have flexibility to choose what works best for their individual property; they may also focus on energy and water conser-vation, use of renewable resources and other issues. Some third-party agencies offer sustainability certifications, and many regional industry associations are working on developing clearer standards.

If you'd like to know if a wine falls into any of these categories, check out the label. Here you'll find a lot of clues—various trademarked symbols and logos are used, and if a winery is going to adhere to these practices, they're likely to want you to know about it. You can also check out a winery's website, which usually goes into details about how a wine was grown and made.

Source: http://www.winespectator.com/drvinny/show/id/41226

ALCOHOL AND THE RISK OF GOUT

According to a recent Harvard University health update, men who drink alcohol, particularly beer, may double their likelihood of developing gout. Humankind has known about this link between alcohol and gout for ages through anecdotal evidence, but now the results of a medical study verify the connection.

Gout is a form of acute arthritis marked by severe pain and inflammation in the joints, particularly the big toe. Episodes of gout strike suddenly without warning. Severe cases of gout may lead to major disability and even kidney failure. More men experience the condition than women, although the difference is less dramatic among the elderly. Researchers believe that while both hereditary and environmental factors lead to gout, environmental causes, such as regular alcohol consumption, are behind the increase in cases of gout in the past thirty years.

The researchers believe beer consumption leads to gout because of its high purine content. Through the process of digestion, the purine compound breaks down to form uric acid. Normally, uric acid leaves the body through urine. But if the kidneys are unable to process all of the uric acid, levels in the blood become too high. The uric acid may then form crystal deposits in the joints. These deposits are the cause of gout.

While powerful medications are available to treat gout, it makes sense to try to lower your risk of developing the disease in the first place. You may be able to ward off gout attacks by avoiding excessive consumption of alcohol and choosing your drink wisely.

Source: http://www.health.harvard.edu/fhg/updates/update0804a.shtml

CHEMICAL ADDITIVES

According to The Center for Science in the Public Interest:

Shopping was easy in the old days, when most U.S. food came from farms. Now, factory-made foods have made chemical additives a significant part of our diet.

Always check food labels and avoid the following ingredients:

- *Sodium nitrite* is a preservative often found in hot dogs, smoked fish and processed meats. It is linked to cancer, especially colon cancer.

- *Saccharin, Aspartame and Acesulfame-K* are artificial sweeteners found in sugar-free desserts, ice cream and soft drinks. Saccharin is linked to cancer in laboratory animals. Aspartame is linked to headaches and is unstable when heated and should not be used in cooking or baking. Acesulfame-K contains a carcinogen that is linked to headaches, nausea and a host of other problems.

- *Caffeine* is found in coffee, tea, guarana, chocolate, cocoa and some energy drinks. It is a nervous system stimulant and can cause insomnia, nervousness, rapid heartbeat, anxiety and hypertension. It acts as a diuretic and can contribute to dehydration.

- *Olestra,* also known as *Olean,* is a fat substitute found in potato chips, crackers and tortilla chips. It is linked to abdominal cramping and diarrhea and decreases absorption of fat-soluble vitamins like A, D, E and K.

- *Food dyes* are found in food, candy, drinks and even toothpastes! They are linked to having an adverse effect on activity and attention in children and may cause cancer.

Source: Center for Science in the Public Interest

For a complete chemical safety guide, visit this website: *http://www.cspinet.org/reports/chemcuisine.htm*

WHY PLATE SIZE MATTERS

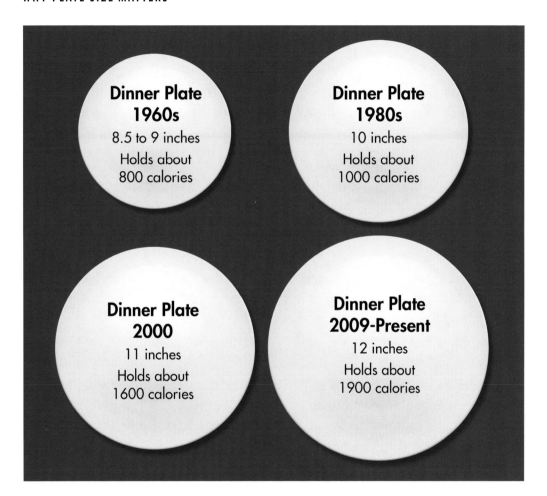

Dinner plate size corresponds with the increase rate of obesity in the U.S. The "see it and eat it" syndrome is a result of falling victim to supersized portions. Europeans tend to eat until they are satisfied and full, and refuse to join the "*Clean Plate Club."

*The Clean Plate Club was a U.S. federal government campaign established in 1917 during World War I to encourage families to finish their entire meal. It was reinstated in 1947 after the Great Depression and World War II. Consuming larger portions compounded with the habit of "cleaning your plate" has led to an obesity and chronic disease epidemic.

RECIPE RULES AND SUBSTITUTIONS

- When a recipe calls for eggs, use large eggs.
- When a recipe calls for almond or soymilk, use original, not vanilla flavor.
- Two egg whites can substitute for one whole egg.
- Always use average-size vegetables unless specified otherwise.
- Carefully wash all fruits and vegetables.
- Use organic, pasture-raised, grass-fed and/or local ingredients whenever available.
- Use natural ingredients without added preservatives, additives or stabilizers.
- Use mostly nonstick pans to cut back on cooking with excess fat.
- Use nonstick olive oil cooking spray or, better yet, wipe a pan with extra-virgin olive oil.
- To reduce fat in baking, replace all or part of the oil/butter with natural applesauce.
- Remove skin before eating poultry.
- For gluten-free breadcrumbs: grind gluten-free oats, flaxseeds or chia seeds and season with herbs.

- Gluten-free grains include amaranth, buckwheat, corn, soy, millet, quinoa, rice, sorghum, teff and wild rice. Oats are inherently gluten-free but are often contaminated with wheat during growing or processing.
- Grains containing gluten: wheat, spelt, kamut, farro, durum, bulgur, semolina, barley, rye and triticale.
- Use more stone-ground cornmeal in baking; it adds a nice flavor. It's available from finely ground to coarsely ground.
- Cut back on the empty calories of *sugar,* also known as corn syrup, high fructose corn syrup, dextrose and sucrose. Use small quantities and stick to more natural forms like pure maple syrup, raw honey, organic blackstrap molasses and organic coconut sugar.

    NOTE: According to MayoClinic.com, giving raw honey to infants may cause infant botulism, a rare but serious gastrointestinal sickness caused by exposure to bacterial spores. Infant botulism can be life-threatening.

- Cut back on salt; it's linked to high blood pressure and should be avoided by those with hypertension, chronic kidney disease or diabetes. Avoid it when you can or use small quantities of sea salt, which is less processed and more flavorful than table salt. Mix sea salt with herbs.

BASIC GUIDE TO MEASURING INGREDIENTS

Make sure you have a set of measuring spoons and cups until you get used to "eyeing" measurements. All measurements should be level. Baking requires accurate measurements of ingredients.

- 1 cup equals 8 fluid ounces or 236.59 milliliters
- 1 fluid ounce equals 2 tablespoons or 29.57 milliliters
- ¼ cup equals 4 tablespoons or 59.15 milliliters
- 3 teaspoons equal one tablespoon or ½ fluid ounce or 14.79 milliliters
- 3 ounces equal the size of the palm of your hand or 85 grams
- 1 ounce equals a 1-inch square (cube) or 28.35 grams
- 2 cups equal 1 pint or 473.18 milliliters
- 4 cups equal 1 quart or 946.36 milliliters (almost one liter)
- 4 cups flour weigh 1 pound or 453.59 grams
- 2 cups milk weigh 1 pound or 453.59 grams
- 4 quarts equal 1 gallon or 3.785 liters

CARLO PETRINI AND THE INTERNATIONAL SLOW FOOD MOVEMENT

Carlo Petrini was born in Bra, Italy, on June 22, 1949. He began writing about wine and food in 1977 and has contributed to hundreds of Italian publications around the world. In 1983, he was instrumental in creating and developing the Italian nonprofit food and wine association, Arcigola.

Frustrated by the industrialization of the food supply and the erosion of quality in the food he saw around him, Petrini began to forge alliances with friends and colleagues with the goals of bringing food back to its roots. In 1986, he founded the International Slow Food Movement as a response to the opening of a McDonald's in Piazza di Spagna in Rome.

He was elected president of the organization at its inception and every year since. Today, the movement exists in over 50 countries and has over 80,000 members and supporters. Slow Food International is responsible for publishing periodicals, books and guides that are read in many languages around the world.

In 2004, Petrini founded a biennial conference called Terra Madre, for which 5,000 small-scale farmers, cooks and food experts gather in Torino, Italy, to share knowledge and build connections.

In addition, every year students from around the globe matriculate at the University of Gastronomic Sciences that Petrini founded in 2004, with campuses in the Italian regions of Piedmont and Emilia-Romagna.

Carlo Petrini is the recipient of many awards and honors, including being named "innovator" in the 2004 Time Magazine list of European heroes. His charisma, passion and conviction are reflected in the popularity of the movement and in the Slow Food philosophy, which seeks a rediscovery of authentic culinary traditions and the pleasures of the table, in addition to the conservation of the world's quality food and wine heritage.

Petrini is a visionary who works to improve the world's agriculture and food supply, one bite at a time.

Source: http://web.princeton.edu/sites/pei/pdf/CarloPetriniBio.pdf

SEAFOOD WATCH: 2013 CULINARY CHART OF ALTERNATIVES

Americans are encouraged to eat local and sustainable seafood, like the Europeans.

Based on where you live in the U.S., use this guide to find ocean-friendly alternatives to seafood on the Seafood Watch "Avoid" list. This information is updated regularly and changes according to scientific findings. The most current information can be found at *www.seafoodwatch.org*.

Avoid	Best Choices	Good Alternatives
Caviar *(Imported Wild)* Caviar: Paddlefish *(US Wild)* Sturgeon *(Imported Wild)*		Caviar: White Sturgeon *(Farmed in Tank Systems in British Columbia, Canada)* Sturgeon: White *(Farmed in Tank Systems in British Columbia, Canada)*

Avoid	Best Choices	Good Alternatives
Chilean Seabass/Patagonian Toothfish *(Crozet Islands, Prince Edward & Marion Islands, Chile)*	Chilean Seabass/ Patagonian Toothfish *(Heard & McDonald Islands, Falkland Islands, Macquarie Island)*	Chilean Seabass/Patagonian Toothfish *(South Georgia, Kerguelen Islands)*
		Chilean Seabass/Antarctic Toothfish *(Ross Sea)*
	Sablefish/Black Cod/ Butterfish *(AK and Canadian Pacific)*	Sablefish/Black Cod/ Butterfish *(CA, OR, WA)*
Cod: Atlantic *(Trawl from Canadian & US Atlantic)*	Cod: Pacific *(Bottom Longline, Jig & Trap from US)*	Cod: Atlantic *(Bottom Gillnet, Bottom Longline, Bottom Trawl and Danish Seine from Iceland & Northeast Arctic)*
Cod: Pacific *(Imported)*	Cod: Atlantic *(Hook-&-Line from Iceland & Northeast Arctic)*	Cod: Atlantic *(US Gulf of Maine Hook-&-Line)*
	Haddock *(US Atlantic Hook-&-Line)*	Cod: Pacific *(US Trawl)*
		Haddock *(Iceland Atlantic & US Atlantic Trawl)*
Crab: Red King *(Russia)*	Crab: Blue *(Trotline from Chesapeake Bay)*	Crab: Blue *(US Pot-caught)*;
	Crab: Dungeness *(CA, OR, WA)*	Crab: Dungeness *(AK)*;
	Crab: Kona *(Australia)*	Crab: Jonah *(US Atlantic)*;
	Crab: Snow *(Eastern Bering Sea, Southern Gulf of St. Lawrence, Canada & US)*	Crab: King *(US)*; Kona *(HI)*;
	Crab: Stone *(US Atlantic and US Gulf of Mexico)*	Crab: Snow *(Eastern Nova Scotia, Newfoundland & Labrador, Canada)*

253

Avoid	Best Choices	Good Alternatives
Dab: Common (Iceland Danish Seine)	Cobia (US Farmed) Halibut: Pacific (US)	Flounder, Sanddab, Sole (US Pacific Wild)
Flounder: Windowpane (US Georges Bank & Gulf of Mexico Bottom Trawl)		Flounder: Summer and Winter (US Atlantic Bottom Trawl)
Flounder: Witch (US Atlantic Bottom Trawl)		Flounder: Windowpane (Bottom Trawl from US Southern New England and US Mid-Atlantic)
Flounder: Yellowtail (US Georges Bank and US Gulf of Mexico Bottom Trawl & Bottom Gillnet)		Halibut: Atlantic (Farmed in Tank Systems in Nova Scotia, Canada)
Flounder: Winter (Bottom Gillnet)		Halibut: California (Hook-&-Line and Bottom Trawl from US Pacific)
Halibut: Atlantic (Bottom Trawl)		Plaice: American (US Atlantic)
Halibut: California (Set Gillnet)		Turbot: Greenland (Canadian Pacific & US Wild)
Grouper (US Atlantic) Grouper: Gag; Snowy; Warsaw; Yellowedge (US Gulf of Mexico)	Mahi Mahi (US Atlantic Troll, Pole) Striped Bass (US Farmed & US Atlantic Hook-&-line)	Black Sea Bass (wild) Grouper: Black & Red (US Gulf of Mexico) Mahi Mahi (US Wild and Imported Troll, Pole) Striped Bass (US Atlantic Gillnet & Pound net)
Hake: White	Tilapia (Farmed in Ecuador & US) Tilapia (Farmed in Tank systems in Canada)	Hake: Offshore, Red & Silver Tilapia (Farmed in China & Taiwan)
Lobster: Caribbean Spiny (Brazil) Lobster: American (Pot and Trap-caught in US Southern New England)	Lobster: California Spiny (CA) Lobster: Caribbean Spiny (FL) Lobster: Spiny (Baja California, Mexico)	Lobster: American (Pot and Trap-caught in US Gulf of Maine, US Georges Bank) Lobster: Caribbean Spiny (Bahamas)
Mahi Mahi (Imported Longline)	Mahi Mahi (US Atlantic Troll, Pole)	Mahi Mahi (US Wild and Imported Troll, Pole)

Avoid	Best Choices	Good Alternatives
Marlin: Blue *(Imported)* Marlin: Striped *(Worldwide)*	Swordfish *(Harpoon & Handline-caught from Canada, US, North Atlantic & East Pacific)*	Marlin: Blue *(HI Wild)* Swordfish *(CA Drift Gillnet)* Swordfish *(HI wild & US Atlantic Longline)*
Orange Roughy	Catfish *(US Farmed)* Tilapia *(Farmed in Ecuador & US)* Tilapia *(Farmed in Tank systems in Canada)*	Flounder: Pacific *(US Pacific Wild)* Flounder: Summer *(US Atlantic Wild)* Tilapia *(Farmed in China & Taiwan)*
Rockfish: Pacific *(Trawl)*	Rockfish: Black *(CA, OR, WA Hook-&-Line)* Sablefish/Black Cod/Butterfish *(AK and Canadian Pacific)* Striped Bass *(US Farmed & US Atlantic Hook-&-line)*	Rockfish *(Pacific Hook-&-Line & Jig)* Sablefish/Black Cod/Butterfish *(CA, OR, WA)* Striped Bass *(US Atlantic Gillnet & Pound net)*
Salmon: Atlantic *(Farmed)*	Arctic Char *(Farmed in Recirculating Systems)* Salmon *(Drift Gillnet, Purse Seine & Troll from AK)* Salmon: Freshwater Coho *(US Farmed in Tank Systems)*	Salmon *(Drift Gillnet, Purse Seine & Troll from CA, OR, WA)* Salmon: Coho *(Canadian Pacific Wild)*
Sharks	Swordfish *(Harpoon & Handline-caught from Canada, US, North Atlantic & East Pacific)* Sturgeon: White *(Farmed in Tank Systems in British Columbia, Canada)*	Sharks: Common Thresher & Shortfin Mako *(Wild from CA & HI)* Sturgeon *(US Farmed)* Sturgeon: White *(OR & WA Wild)* Swordfish *(CA Drift Gillnet)* Swordfish *(HI wild & US Atlantic Longline)*

255

Avoid	Best Choices	Good Alternatives
Shrimp *(Imported)*	Prawn: Spot *(Canadian Pacific)* Shrimp *(US Farmed in Fully Recirculating Systems or Inland Ponds)* Shrimp: Black Tiger *(Farmed using Selva Shrimp® Criteria in Ca Mau Province of Southern Vietnam & other areas of Southeast Asia,)* Shrimp: Pink *(OR)*	Prawn: Spot *(US Pacific)* Shrimp *(Wild from Canada & US)* Shrimp *(US Farmed in Open Systems)* Shrimp *(Thailand farmed in Fully Recirculating Systems)*
Snapper: Red *(Imported & US Gulf of Mexico)* Snapper: Vermilion *(US)*	Tilapia *(Farmed in Ecuador & US)* Tilapia *(Farmed in Tank systems in Canada)*	Snapper: Gray; Lane; Mutton; Yellowtail *(Wild from US Atlantic & US Gulf of Mexico)* Snapper: Gray; Pink; Red; Ruby *(HI Wild)* Snapper: Silk *(Wild from US Caribbean, US Gulf of Mexico & US South Atlantic)* Tilapia *(Farmed in China & Taiwan)*
Swordfish *(Imported)*	Mahi Mahi *(US Atlantic Troll, Pole)* Swordfish *(Harpoon & Handline-caught from Canada, US, North Atlantic & East Pacific)*	Mahi Mahi *(US Wild and Imported Troll, Pole)* Swordfish *(CA Drift Gillnet)* Swordfish *(HI wild & US Atlantic Longline)*
Tilefish: Blueline & Golden *(US Gulf of Mexico & US South Atlantic)*	Mahi Mahi *(US Atlantic Troll, Pole)* Striped Bass *(US Farmed & US Atlantic Hook-&-line)*	Mahi Mahi *(US Wild and Imported Troll, Pole)* Tilefish: Golden *(US Mid-Atlantic)* Striped Bass *(US Atlantic Gillnet & Pound net)*

Avoid	Best Choices	Good Alternatives
Tuna: Canned	Tuna: "White" Canned Albacore *(Troll, Pole from Canadian & US Pacific)* Tuna: "Light" Canned Skipjack *(Troll, Pole)*	Tuna: "White" Canned Albacore *(Troll, Pole except Canadian & US Pacific)*
Tuna: Albacore *(North Atlantic & All Longline except HI)* Tuna: Bigeye *(All Longline except US Atlantic)* Tuna: Blackfin *(All Longline & Purse Seine)* Tuna: Bluefin *(Wild or Ranched)* Tuna: Skipjack *(Purse Seine & All Imported Longline)* Tuna: Tongol *(All Gillnet & Purse Seine except Malaysia)* Tuna: Yellowfin *(All Purse Seine & Longline except HI & US Atlantic)*	Tuna: Albacore *(Troll, Pole from Canadian & US Pacific)* Tuna: Bigeye *(Troll, Pole from US Atlantic)* Tuna: Skipjack *(Troll, Pole)* Tuna: Yellowfin *(Troll, Pole from Pacific & US Atlantic)*	Tuna: Albacore *(HI Longline & South Atlantic Troll, Pole)* Tuna: Bigeye *(Troll, Pole & US Atlantic Longline)* Tuna: Blackfin *(Troll, Pole)* Tuna: Skipjack *(HI & US Atlantic Longline)* Tuna: Tongol *(Troll, Pole or from Malaysia)* Tuna: Yellowfin *(Troll, Pole Except Pacific & US Atlantic)* Tuna: Yellowfin *(HI & US Atlantic Longline)*

Key

AK: Alaska

CA: California

FL: Florida

HI: Hawaii

OR: Oregon

WA: Washington

Mid-Atlantic: New York to North Carolina

Northeast: Connecticut to Maine

Southeast: South Carolina to Texas

/ A slash is used to separate different market names for the same fish.

Courtesy of Monterey Bay Aquarium

257

SHOPPER'S GUIDE TO PESTICIDES IN PRODUCE, 2013

In the U.S., the following 15 fruits and vegetables had the *highest* pesticide load. That's why it's so important to buy organically grown produce whenever it's available.

Apples	Potatoes
Celery	Spinach
Cherry tomatoes	Strawberries
Cucumbers	Sweet bell peppers
Grapes	Collard greens
Hot peppers	Kale
Nectarines (imported)	Summer squash & zucchini
Peaches	

In the U.S., the following produce items were found to have the *lowest* residual pesticide load, making them the safest choices among conventionally grown produce:

Asparagus	Kiwi
Avocado	Mango
Cabbage	Mushrooms
Cantaloupe	Onions
Sweet corn (choose non-GMO)	Eggplant
Papayas (choose non-GMO*)	Pineapple
*Most Hawaiian papaya is GMO)	Sweet peas (frozen)
Grapefruit	Sweet potatoes

Source: The Environmental Working Group

HERB AND SPICE SEASONING GUIDE

There are many herbs and spices commonly used around the world in various combinations. Seasoning is a personal choice, so experiment and create your own blends that tantalize your taste buds! It's a great way to "get off" the saltshaker and enhance the flavor of quality ingredients. The following is a partial list:

Allspice: Lean ground meats, stews, tomatoes, peaches, applesauce, cranberry sauce, gravies, lean meat

Almond extract: Puddings, fruits

Basil: Fish, lamb, lean ground meats, stews, salads, soups, sauces, fish cocktails

Bay leaves: Lean meats, stews, poultry, soups, tomatoes

Black peppercorns: A perfect seasoning for any food

Caraway seeds: Lean meats, stews, soups, salads, breads, cabbage, asparagus, noodles

Chives: Salads, sauces, soups, lean meat dishes, vegetables

Cider vinegar: Salads, vegetables, sauces

Cinnamon: Fruits (especially apples), breads, pie crusts

Curry powder: Lean meats (especially lamb), veal, chicken, fish, tomatoes, tomato soup, mayonnaise

Dill: Fish sauces, soups, tomatoes, cabbage, carrots, cauliflower, green beans, cucumbers, potatoes, salads, macaroni, lean beef, lamb, chicken, fish

Espelette pepper (in place of black pepper): Eggs, sauces, vegetables, sandwiches, potatoes, meats, poultry

Garlic (not garlic salt): Lean meats, fish, soups, salads, vegetables, tomatoes, potatoes

Ginger: Chicken, fruits

Lemon juice: Lean meats, fish, poultry, salads, vegetables

Mace: Hot breads, apples, fruit salads, carrots, cauliflower, squash, potatoes, veal, lamb

Mustard (dry): Lean ground meats, lean meats, chicken, fish, salads, asparagus, broccoli, Brussels sprouts, cabbage, mayonnaise, sauces

Nutmeg: Fruits, pie crust, lemonade, potatoes, chicken, fish, lean meat loaf, toast, veal, pudding

Onion powder (not onion salt): Lean meats, stews, vegetables, salads, soups

Paprika: Lean meats, fish, soups, salads, sauces, vegetables, eggs

Parsley: Lean meats, fish, soups, salads, sauces, vegetables

Peppermint extract: Puddings, fruits

Pimiento: Salads, vegetables, casserole dishes

Pink Peppercorns: Salad dressings, fish, pasta, eggs, poultry, vegetables

Rosemary: Chicken, veal, extra-lean beef, lean pork, sauces, stuffing, potatoes, peas, lima beans

Sage: Lean meats, stews, biscuits, tomatoes, green beans, fish, lima beans, onions, lean pork

Savory: Salads, lean pork, lean ground meats, soups, green beans, squash, tomatoes, lima beans, peas

Sumac: Eggs, salads, meats

Thyme: Lean meats (especially veal and lean pork), sauces, soups, onions, peas, tomatoes, salads

Turmeric: Lean meats, fish, sauces, rice, eggs

White pepper (in place of black pepper when you don't want to see specks of black): mashed potatoes, white sauces and seafood

Sodium chloride or table salt is approximately 40 percent sodium.

The American Heart Association recommends consuming less than 1,500 milligrams (mg) of sodium a day.

¼ teaspoon salt = 600 mg sodium   ½ teaspoon salt = 1,200 mg sodium

¾ teaspoon salt = 1,800 mg sodium   1 teaspoon salt = 2,400 mg sodium

Source: Adapted from The American Heart Association

USDA FOOD PYRAMID (2005)

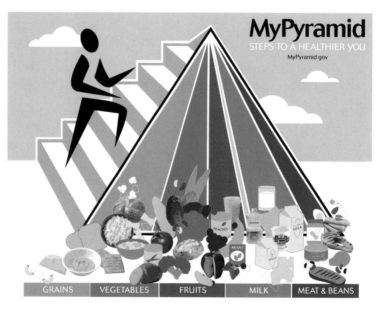

Source: http://www.mypyramid.gov/

USDA 2011 MYPLATE

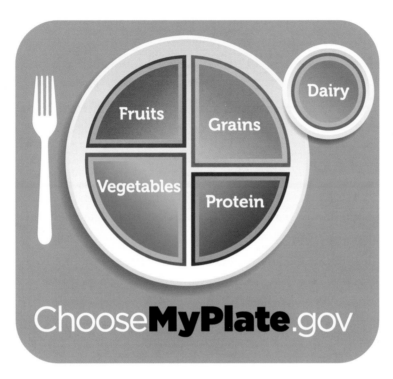

Source: http://www.choosemyplate.gov

WHOLE GRAINS, A TO Z

Amaranth has a high level of complete protein; its protein contains lysine, an amino acid missing or negligible in many grains.

Barley is high in soluble fiber and may lower cholesterol even more effectively than oat fiber.

Buckwheat, not a wheat, is the only grain known to have high levels of the antioxidant rutin, and studies show that it improves circulation and prevents LDL cholesterol from blocking blood vessels.

Bulgur, cracked wheat, has more fiber than quinoa, oats, millet, buckwheat or corn. Its quick cooking time and mild flavor make it ideal for those new to whole-grains.

Corn has the highest level of antioxidants of any grain or vegetable—almost twice the antioxidant activity of apples!

Farro, also called emmer, is an ancient strain of wheat. Semolina flour, made from emmer, is used for special soups and dishes in Tuscany and Umbria, and is thought by some aficionados to make the best pasta.

Kamut, an heirloom grain, has higher levels of protein than common wheat, and more vitamin E.

Millet, a staple in India is a tiny grain with a mild flavor.

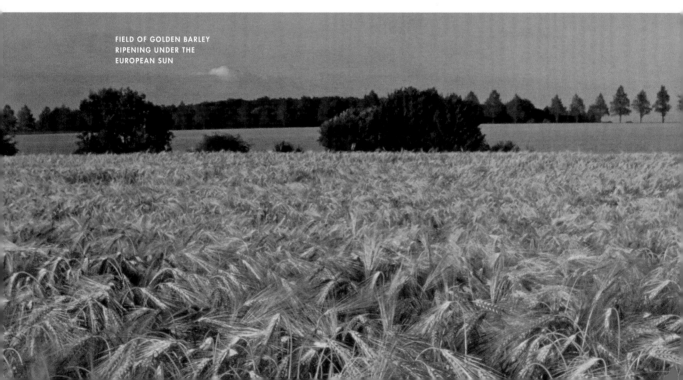

FIELD OF GOLDEN BARLEY RIPENING UNDER THE EUROPEAN SUN

Oats (like barley) contain a fiber called beta-glucan known to lower cholesterol; they also contain a unique antioxidant known to protect blood vessels from LDL cholesterol.

Quinoa is a complete protein with all essential amino acids.

Rice is one of the most easily digested grains—one reason rice cereal is often recommended as a baby's first solid food; rice is also ideal for those on a gluten-free diet.

Rye contains a type of fiber that promotes a rapid feeling of fullness, so it's a good choice for people trying to lose weight.

Sorghum, also called milo, is a gluten-free grain and popular in the celiac diet.

Spelt is a variety of wheat and is higher in protein than common wheat.

Teff has over twice the iron of other grains and three times the calcium.

Triticale, a hybrid between durum wheat and rye, is mostly grown in Europe without fertilizers and pesticides.

Wheat is high in gluten. Besides being popular in pasta and bread, it can be cracked (bulgur) or cooked whole (wheat berries).

Wild rice is not rice, but the seed of a grass. It has twice the protein and fiber of brown rice, but less iron and calcium.

263

Source: Excerpt from Whole Grains, A to Z, courtesy of Oldways Preservation Trust and the Whole Grains Council, www.wholegrainscouncil.org

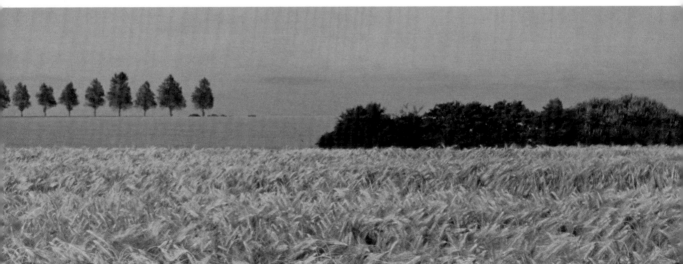

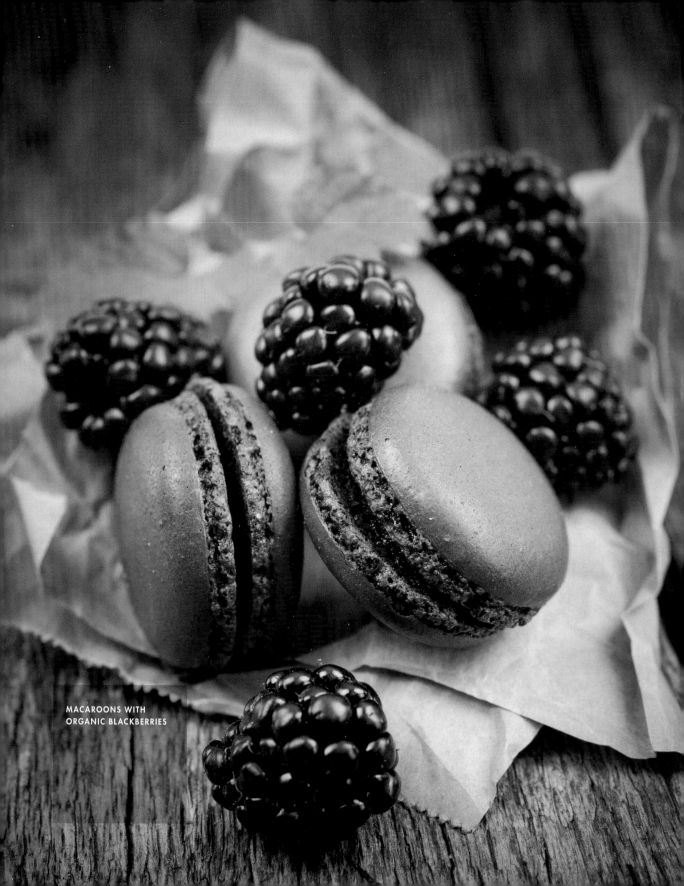

MACAROONS WITH
ORGANIC BLACKBERRIES

INDEX

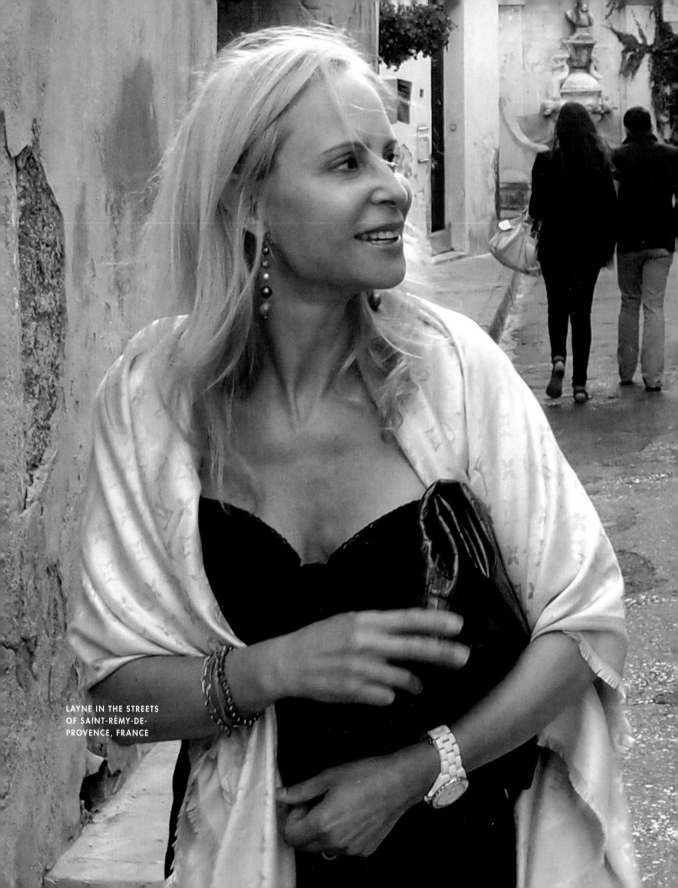

LAYNE IN THE STREETS OF SAINT-RÉMY-DE-PROVENCE, FRANCE

ACKNOWLEDGMENTS

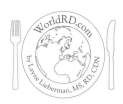

Every major event during my professional career has brought me new growth and awareness—but the experience of writing this book has been in a class by itself! I could not have done it without my husband, Michael Liebelson, and my editor, Claire Gerus.

Michael traveled with me by train, automobile and plane to food markets, outdoor markets, shops, halls, restaurants, cafés, farms, and vineyards throughout France, Italy, Switzerland and other countries. He put up with my long, late hours as I hovered over my laptop and satisfied my compulsion to photograph food at *every* opportunity. He is truly my number one!

I am grateful to Claire Gerus for being an inspiration and believing that I could make this dream happen. Claire is the most devoted and talented editor one could wish for, and I'm so lucky to have had her in my life for the past two years. She has been my guiding light and advisor, spending endless hours through multiple time zones helping me get to this grand finale! Because I knew that Claire would be there when I needed her, I never gave up, and for that I love her dearly.

You know the saying, "It takes a village to raise a child—and to publish a book!" While writing a book requires endless "alone" hours, mostly productive but sometimes sidetracked, this journey took me not only across the world, but deep into my heart. I wish to thank the following very special people who helped me make this book a reality: Bill Greaves, Len Riggio, Diane Simowski, Chef Aviva Wolf (my professional recipe tester and who also shot a few of the food photographs), Amy Collins, Julie Ballou, Michele DeFilippo, Ronda Rawlins, Betsy Thorpe and Claudia Uscategui.

Bill Greaves is a brilliant graphic designer, a blend of talent, creativity and a fantastic British sense of humor. I was also grateful to have Bill's male perspective on dietary matters, and his European flair was invaluable!

Thank you to the following European friends, acquaintances and devoted chefs who made time to share their thoughts, perspectives and insights. Every one of them helped shape this book (in alphabetical order): Elena Arzak, Paul Bocuse, Christian Étienne, Tanja Grandit, Rolf Hiltl, Sophie Lyonnet, Alessandro Negrini, Nadia Perna, Fabio Pisani, Pedro Subijana, Christian Tetedoie and Matthiew Viannay.

269

While moving through the creative process that produced *Beyond the Mediterranean Diet: European Secrets of the Super-Healthy*, I recalled the many wonderful people who have influenced my career and life. Because of you, my horizons have been expanded and my perspectives have broadened. Without you, I would not be where I am today. Thank you (in alphabetical order) to: Alexander F. Anapol, Benjamin H. Anapol (photo credit for yogurt panna cotta), Irma Anapol, Starr Boggs, Dana Conklin, Thomas Cullen, John Gambino, Dr. Judith Gilbride, Melanie Kaye-Melia, Bea Lewis, Loretta and David Lieberman, Chef Frank Lucas, Dr. Robert Parker, Leatrice Spanierman and Dr. Judith Wylie-Rosett.

Danke, grazie, merci and thank you to anyone else who offered support, guidance and just plain love.

Thank you all so much for being a part of this amazing journey!

270

INSIDE COVER COLLAGES

Inside cover collages show gourmands and acclaimed chefs who share a passion for fine food and use the highest-quality local ingredients.

Inside front cover photos include (in alphabetical order):
Elena Arzak of Restaurant Arzak, San Sebastián, Spain
Starr Boggs of Starr Boggs Restaurant, Westhampton Beach, New York
John Gambino of Baby Moon Restaurant, Westhampton Beach, New York
Eric Kayser of Maison Kayser Bakeries, Paris, France and New York, New York
Frank Lucas of Starr Boggs Restaurant, Westhampton Beach, New York
Pepa Muñoz of El Qüenco de Pepa, Madrid, Spain
Alessandro Negrini and Pisano Fabio of Il Luogo di Aimo e Nadia, Milan, Italy

Inside back cover photos include (in alphabetical order):
Graeme Cheevers of Martin Wishart at Loch Lomond, Alexandria, Scotland
Philippe Chevrier of Domaine de Chateauvieux, Satigny-Genève, Switzerland
Member of Private Men's Cooking Club, San Sebastián, Spain
Tanja Grandits of Restaurant Stucki, Basel, Switzerland
Maya Gurley of Maya's Restaurant, Saint Barthélemy, French West Indies
Pascual and Marisa Adan Millan and Family, Zaragoza, Spain
Pedro Subijana and Itsasne Markaide of Restaurant Akelarre, San Sebastián, Spain